Cope With
Infertility

Hodder Arnold

A MEMBER OF THE HODDER HEADLINE GROUP

Cope With
Infertility

Claire Gillman
Edited by Denise Robertson

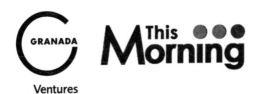

Ventures

Hodder Arnold

A MEMBER OF THE HODDER HEADLINE GROUP

Orders: Please contact Bookpoint Ltd, 130 Milton Park, Abingdon, Oxon OX14 4SB. Telephone: +44 (0) 1235 827720. Fax: +44 (0) 1235 400454. Lines are open 09.00 to 5.00, Monday to Saturday, with a 24-hour message answering service. You can also order through our website www.hoddereducation.co.uk.

British Library Cataloguing in Publication Data
A catalogue record for this title is available from the British Library.

ISBN-13: 978 0 340 94323 6

First published   2007
Impression number 10 9 8 7 6 5 4 3 2 1
Year   2012 2011 2010 2009 2008 2007

Typeset by Transet Limited, Coventry, England.
Printed in Great Britain for Hodder Education, a division of Hodder Headline, an Hachette Livre UK Company, 338 Euston Road, London, NW1 3BH, by Cox & Wyman Ltd, Reading, Berkshire.

Hodder Headline's policy is to use papers that are natural, renewable and recyclable products and made from wood grown in sustainable forests. The logging and manufacturing processes are expected to conform to the environmental regulations of the country of origin.

ABOUT THE AUTHORS

Claire Gillman is an experienced journalist and writer who regularly contributes to national newspapers and magazines. She's a former magazine editor on titles including *Health & Fitness* and *Girl About Town*. Claire has written eight adult health and parenting books, and six children's books under the pen-name of Rory Storm.

Denise Robertson's television career began with *BBC Breakfast Time* in 1984. She has been the resident agony aunt of ITV's *This Morning* for the last 20 years. In that time she has received over 200,000 letters covering a wide range of problems from viewers and from readers of her newspaper and magazine columns. She has written 19 novels and several works of non-fiction. Her autobiography, *Agony: Don't Get Me Started,* was published in paperback by Little Books in July 2007. She is associated with many charities, among them Relate, The Bubble Foundation, Careline and the National Council for the Divorced and Separated.

WHICH PAGE?

CONTENTS

FOREWORD

By Fern Britton and Phillip Schofield

As presenters of ITV's *This Morning*, over many years we have met many incredible people with many incredible stories to tell. What we have learnt is that life can be wonderful but it can also be very hard.

Our phone-ins have generated thousands of calls a day from viewers all over Great Britain looking for suitable advice on a range of subjects. What is very obvious from these calls is that we are not alone with the personal challenges we often face and there is a great need for help in dealing with them. We are always cheered by the follow-up letters and emails from viewers saying how our experts' advice has helped them to turn their lives around.

Over the 20 years *This Morning* has been on air, Denise Robertson, our agony aunt, has regularly offered support and advice to millions of viewers on a huge range of personal problems and she spends even more time off-screen answering letters, calling those in distress and dealing with questions via the internet. As a result she is uniquely qualified to edit these books which reflect the common sense and sensitive advice that we provide on the show.

We believe these survival guides will help you to deal with the practical and emotional fallout caused by issues such as bereavement, relationship break-ups, debt, infertility, addiction, domestic violence and depression.

If you feel that your particular problems are insurmountable – don't! There is always a way to improve your life or at least get yourself on a path towards a new start. If you think you are alone with your problem – don't! Our experience shows that many of us all face the same problems but are often reluctant to admit it. You have already made a great start by picking up this book.

We both wish you all the strength and support you need to tackle your own personal problems and sincerely hope that we can help through these books and through our continued work on the programme.

INTRODUCTION

Most of us, if we want to have children, take giving birth for granted. One day, when we're ready, we know it will happen. The idea of reproduction as a right is so deep-seated that the possibility that we could be infertile comes as a nasty shock. Yet infertility affects about 15 per cent of couples of childbearing age. And it is not just a woman's concern; a problem with the man is the sole or a contributing cause of infertility in about half of infertile couples, and about one-third of infertile couples have more than one cause or factor related to their inability to conceive. Nearly one-fifth of couples have no identifiable cause for their infertility.

The good news is that help is available. For some, it will be a relatively simple process to encourage conception. Others may have to resort to the more sophisticated techniques available today. For most couples, their journey into the world of fertility treatment will end in a live birth. For those few who face eventual disappointment, there are other options.

This book is written for everyone who fears that infertility may be a problem, for those undergoing treatment, and for the few who must seek alternative means of starting a family. Our aim is to offer information that will help you to make choices along the way.

Infertility treatment is available to everyone in the UK, and people working in the field are skilled and sympathetic to their patients' needs. However, it is still helpful to gather as much information as you can before you embark on treatment. We've tried to give the facts in an easy to understand manner and to offer help not only to those setting out in trepidation but to others who may have grown weary of the regime they have to follow to achieve the desired result. We also discuss the options available if you eventually decide that you do not wish to proceed with treatment. This book is written to help both men and women because infertility is a problem for men and women alike.

Whatever your choice about the way ahead, we hope this book helps you to achieve a satisfactory ending to your story.

Denise Robertson

Part 1:
What to Do
Right Now

1

Help is at hand

If you suspect or know that you have infertility issues, you are probably feeling very alone and isolated right now. In fact, you may be reading this book because you feel unable to speak to family and friends about your emotions or to discuss what you're going through.

When friends and contemporaries all appear to be starting a family and people around you take having a baby for granted, as a natural progression of life if you like, then struggling to conceive can make you feel extremely lonely and excluded.

Yet, rest assured, **you are not alone**. An astonishing one in six couples seeks specialist help at some time in their lives because of the difficulty of conceiving. If that fact is small consolation to you, the better news is that there is an enormous array of information and expert advice as well as self-help, complementary and medical treatments now available that can vastly improve your chances of having a baby.

Even for those couples with perfect reproductive health and with no fertility problems, it can take longer than you might think to become pregnant. On average, one couple in every five will not conceive in the first year of trying.

However, we understand how worried you may feel if you find yourself in this one-in-five category, or if you've been trying for a much-wanted baby for even longer than a year. It is only natural to be concerned and anxious, but try not to worry too much – help is at hand.

How this book can help you

You have taken the first vital step on the path through this perplexing, frustrating and upsetting period in your life by reading this book. Armed with the information and advice it contains, you will have a better idea of where to go for further help and how best to get through this testing time and achieve a positive outcome.

Irrespective of whether a problem lies with you or your partner, or whether there is no apparent reason why you haven't become pregnant so far, it is worth bearing in mind that, for most couples, there is always something that can be done to improve the chances of conceiving a healthy baby either naturally or using assisted techniques. These range from drug treatments through complementary and alternative therapies to medical techniques such as IVF (in vitro

Q. We've been trying to conceive for eight months. Is there something wrong?

A. It's perfectly normal for healthy, fertile couples to take months and even a year or more to conceive. Of course, you can visit your doctor to discuss your concerns but it is early days to be unduly worried. Try not to be anxious, but don't leave it too much longer without consulting your doctor.

fertilization). We'll go through these options with you in a simple, step-by-step way so that you are confident about what is right for you and happy in the choices that you make.

In Chapter 2, we offer advice on how to deal with the roller-coaster of emotions that you are going through and suggest some practical guidance on getting through the days and weeks ahead in as relaxed and positive a way as possible. There are also tips for reducing the painful awareness of your problem that you may be experiencing at the moment plus quick-fix methods to boost your self-confidence in situations where you feel vulnerable and uncomfortable.

We look at ways to inter-react with members of your family, friends and the world in general, and we recommend ways for you and your partner to help each other through what can be a painful and distressing time for you both.

In addition, there is also a whole host of professional services and support groups available (populated with people who are going through the same experiences as yourself), if you feel the need to speak to someone in confidence from outside your circle of friends and family.

Before we come to the advice on recognizing and getting through the emotions that you are experiencing right now, let's look at some of the facts behind infertility. We will attempt to demystify some of the confusing language and terminology that surrounds this emotive subject.

MYTH: It's usually the woman who has the infertility problem.

FACT: In couples that are experiencing difficulty trying to conceive, the problem lies equally with both the man and the woman, with both female and male factors accounting for 40 per cent of infertile couples. Sometimes the cause is unknown and occasionally it is a combination of the two individuals that creates a problem. Irrespective of who may be the cause medically, it is unhelpful to point the finger of blame, especially since both of you are in this together, and it is a shared problem.

What is infertility?

Unless you have a medical background, you are now entering into a world in which you are probably completely unfamiliar. If you've had a chance to check out any websites or literature on the subject of infertility, you'll realize that the whole topic is couched in confusing and unfamiliar terms and phrases. Don't be put off by the jargon though. It is simply a way for health professionals to classify the particular problems you may be facing, and to recognize your present situation so that they know how to help you to achieve a healthy pregnancy.

Nonetheless, a bit of insider knowledge can be a useful thing. Overleaf is a breakdown of the terms used to describe the state of your reproductive health (in layman's terms, how likely you are to conceive), and their meanings.

MYTH: You are a failure as a woman if you cannot produce a child.

FACT: Giving birth does not make someone a success, nor does being unable to have a baby make you a failure in any way. Never lose sight of that fact.

Fertile: You are fully capable of conceiving and sustaining a pregnancy. Although men and women who are fertile should be able to conceive naturally and without difficulty, this has no bearing on the length of time it may take to get pregnant. Even the most fertile couples do not always conceive on the first or even the second or third attempt – it takes many healthy couples over a year.

Sub-fertile: This is the term given to those couples who have a reduced ability to conceive. It describes those people who have obstacles to getting pregnant but, in the majority of cases, these problems are solved relatively easily.

Infertile: If you have been having unprotected sex for over 12 months (six months if you are a woman over 35 years old) without conceiving naturally, then you are considered infertile by the medical profession. Although the term itself sounds like a terrifyingly final and permanent verdict, being classed as 'infertile' does not mean that you will never have a child. It simply means that you are unlikely to do so without taking certain measures or without medical intervention.

Confusing though it sounds, your doctor may also refer to you as being infertile if you are able to get pregnant but unable to carry pregnancies to full term (to deliver your baby after nine months).

Secondary infertility: If you already have a child but have problems conceiving second or subsequent children, you could be described as having secondary infertility.

Zero fertility: Although relatively rare, this is the term given to those with a serious and occasionally insurmountable problem, such as blocked tubes in a woman or lack of sperm in a man, in which case you will be unable to conceive naturally. Nonetheless, although this is a serious diagnosis, remember that you may still be able to conceive with the help of medical or surgical intervention.

Two-minute relaxation exercise

Stress and tension are one of your biggest enemies when you are trying to get pregnant. So, before you embark on any programme of investigations, testing or treatment, get into the habit of running through this simple relaxation routine several times a day.

You'll be shocked at just how tense you have become, and astonished at how much more relaxed you feel in body and mind after just two minutes!

1 Close your eyes and breathe in deeply.

2 Consciously relax your muscles, dropping your shoulders, uncreasing your furrowed brow, and unclenching your hands.

3 Now, as you breathe in through your nose, count for six (if you are happy with visualization, try seeing the incoming breath as a beautiful bright blue colour).

4 Hold for a count of four.

5 Gently breathe out, this time through your mouth for a count of six (again, for those who

are comfortable with visualization, imagine your exhaled breath is the colour of gold).

6 Repeat three times.

Wow, you're feeling more relaxed already, aren't you? Practise this simple exercise whenever you feel yourself getting tense, or your emotions are threatening to overwhelm you, and you'll be amazed at how much more relaxed and in control you feel.

How do you know if you're infertile?

The very fact that you are reading this book suggests that, at the very least, you are concerned about the time it is taking to conceive, and you may suspect that you are facing fertility issues. Perhaps you harbour a suspicion that your partner's fertility is not as high as it could be. It often takes some months of trying before even the most fertile of couples can conceive a child (seven months is the UK national average), so possibly you should not be worrying just yet, hard though it may be to stop.

It's easy for us to say, we know, but at this early stage you should try to relax (see page 12 as well as find further suggestions for relaxation techniques in Chapter 2). Don't forget to enjoy your lives together as a couple, and let 'trying for a baby' be a natural part of your life rather than the focus of it. However, if your suspicions persist and with each passing month you become more disappointed as you realize that you are not pregnant, then you should go to see your doctor without delay.

That said, although your doctor will be happy to discuss your concerns and give advice on what tests might be appropriate, if you are under 35 years of age, your doctor will not put you forward for fertility testing until you have been having unprotected sex for at least a year and are still not pregnant. This timescale drops for women over 35 – you are advised to start investigations after six months of unprotected sex without a pregnancy. But don't panic: this doesn't mean that time has run out. Rather that it is prudent to identify any problems as early as possible.

Unfortunately, without test results, it is impossible to confirm for sure whether you are fully fertile and simply experiencing a delay in conceiving a baby, or whether you and/or your partner have sub-fertility or infertility issues.

Of course, it may be that you have already started down this route and that your doctor has run some tests and you are now having to face the fact that your longed-for baby is not going to happen automatically.

Wherever you find yourself on this spectrum, we understand what a worrying and upsetting time this is for you. It is tough when you don't know if you have a problem or not, and it is of course even more difficult to have your fears confirmed and to find out that your chances of conceiving naturally are reduced.

Whether you are worried about your fertility or know for sure that you have problems to overcome, don't lose sight of the fact that there's still hope. With all the help and advice that is now available and the advances in modern medical practices, the chances of having a baby for couples experiencing fertility problems has improved immeasurably. And you have taken a huge stride closer to achieving your goal because you are actively doing something about it and seeking help.

MYTH: Your chances of getting pregnant after having an abortion are reduced.

FACT: An abortion does not affect a woman's future fertility. In the past, when abortions were illegal, operations were performed in back streets using unsterilized equipment and dangerous techniques. As a result, complications were common and ensuing infections could lead to infertility. Operations are now carried out in sterile hospital environments and fertility should not be affected. If you have had an abortion in the past, do not beat yourself up or blame yourself for your current difficulties in conceiving. This is not a judgement and the two are almost certainly not linked.

How you are feeling right now

A diagnosis of infertility can have a devastating impact on your lives. There seem to be so many obstacles to overcome before you can even reach the stage of having treatment, let alone reaching the holy grail of finding out that you are expecting a long-awaited baby. Even a delay in getting pregnant of several months can be upsetting and frustrating, and it is common for couples to start to worry, despite assurances that there is no need to panic at this early stage.

In Chapter 2, we explore in depth the range of emotions that you and your loved ones might experience as you go through the processes of dealing with delayed conception or infertility, and we give you practical advice on how to handle these feelings effectively.

Right now you may be experiencing some of the most common reactions and emotions that couples express when they first discover that they may have problems in getting pregnant. Whether you recognize some or all of them, it's worth bearing in mind that they are all perfectly natural and legitimate reactions to the position you find yourself in and that there are effective techniques that you can use to deal with them.

Fear: Will treatment work? Fear of failure. Fear of a future without children.

Anger: 'Why me?' is a common reaction, often accompanied by anger towards the 'experts' ('Why can't they treat me?'), towards society ('Why didn't they warn me about infertility'), and towards your partner who is a constant reminder of your mutual failure to conceive.

Resentment: It seems so unfair that some parents neglect or don't make the most of their children when you know that you and your partner will make a loving, attentive mum and dad.

Shock: 'Is this really happening to me?' can be swiftly followed by numbness and withdrawal, or in some cases, denial.

Guilt: 'It's something I did. This is my fault.' Sadly, this is an all too common reaction, but it is not your fault.

Shame: Feeling that you have let down your partner and loved ones.

Confusion: Trying to decide what is the right course of action for you and making the right choices about treatment is very bewildering. No wonder you feel lost and confused.

Exhaustion: It is extremely draining to live with the overwhelming desire for a family, and to experience the desolation of loss and failure when you can't conceive.

Panic: 'I've left it too late and time has run out.' This is particularly common in career women who have left it until their thirties to start a family, and it can lead to a rising panic that threatens to overrun all aspects of your life.

Isolation: Many couples experiencing infertility confess to feeling on the fringe of life and that they cannot fully participate in society. 'Everyone is normal and has a family except me', is a common and extremely destructive feeling.

Impotence: All of the above reactions to your situation and the sheer power of your emotions can leave you feeling hopeless and helpless. But remember, you've done the right thing – you have reached for the help of this book.

Q. I feel like I'm the only person in the world who is having problems conceiving. Is it normal to feel so alone?

A. Many couples experiencing fertility problems describe feeling isolated and alone but having trouble becoming pregnant is really not that unusual. The chances are that you will know someone in your circle of friends and family who is going through or has gone through the same experience as yourself. It is just that people don't tend to talk about it. Rest assured, you are not alone and, if you think it would be beneficial to talk to someone who is in a similar situation, there is bound to be a local support group who can help (see Part 5, Chapter 12 for details).

Q. Can I sort this out for myself? Do I have to involve medical professionals?

A. There is a great deal that you can do yourself to improve your fertility and raise your chances of conceiving naturally, as we'll discuss in Chapter 4.

Nonetheless, there may be an underlying reason for your inability to conceive and this may have to be identified and rectified by medical professionals. So, while it is a great idea to take every step possible to help yourself and to aim for optimum health, in general it is still advisable to seek professional help and advice.

Why me?

As you mentally tick off some or all of the emotions on the list on pages 18 and 19, you may be feeling pretty dejected and low at this point. All this has probably come as such a surprise to you. For most of us, it never crosses our mind that there might be problems when the time comes to start a family. In this day and age, where we have the lives and careers we choose and we dictate our own lifestyles, it comes as a shock to find that the thing you want most in life is being denied to you. And it is so unfair. If you have always been an organized person, able to make decisions and holding down a responsible job, it is very hard to find yourself in a situation that you cannot fully control. We understand this, but you can do something, and **you can start right now**.

Don't worry: You are on the right path

We know that you may be feeling desolate and discouraged at the moment and we fully acknowledge the pain you are experiencing if you have been told that you may not be able to have a family. But please don't despair. There is so much that you and your partner can do to make things better, to optimize your physical and emotional well-being and to improve your chances of a successful pregnancy. We promise to help you along the path to this brighter future and to an outcome that you can be truly happy about.

We recommend that you take your time to read and digest each chapter of the book and you will then be able to cherry-pick the advice and information that suits your particular situation.

In my heart of hearts, I knew we had a problem but I was scared to do anything about it. It was torture, but I preferred living in hope each month, only to have my hopes dashed when my period came, than being told by the experts that we couldn't have a baby on our own.

Eventually, I felt like I was losing my mind and I was so desperate that I went to the doctor. He ran tests and, sure enough, Mark had a low sperm count. We were amazed at how straightforward the treatment was for us. Our son is now six months old, and I only wish I'd asked for help sooner.

Julie

It took me ten years of trying to conceive before I finally gave birth to a healthy baby girl. We had several different treatments and so many losses and I'll never forget how empty I felt through that time, even though my world has now been transformed by my beautiful daughter.

Angela

2

Emotional strategies

Some people seem to be able to accept delays and difficulties in becoming pregnant calmly and with poise, but the majority find the fear of infertility deeply distressing. Many couples experience a rollercoaster of emotions, ranging from disbelief, anger and frustration to guilt, despondency and despair.

Although all these emotions are perfectly legitimate, they can occasionally overwhelm you to the extent that sometimes you hardly recognize yourself. At these times, it's easy to forget that you are a confident, self-assured, happy and positive person. Don't worry, many women experience these feelings of insecurity when they are waiting to become pregnant, but they are fleeting, and as you become clearer about what is happening to you and how you plan to handle your fertility experience, so you will get the old, carefree you back.

The aim of this chapter is to help you to identify what you and your partner might be experiencing emotionally at the moment and to give you strategies to allow you to cope with these powerful feelings. There is also some practical advice on how best to deal with family and friends and, equally important for some people, how to face up to a world that doesn't seem to understand what you are going through.

How can you get through this?

The frustration and upset of delayed pregnancy very often leads to emotions such as anger, resentment, jealousy and frustration – emotions that you may not be used to but that are perfectly normal, so try not to worry unduly on that score. While it is normal to feel this way and to acknowledge your feelings, you should also realize that **your emotional state has a strong influence on your physical health**, and stress and negative emotions can affect you and your partner's fertility for the worse.

So, although we know it's not easy, it is important that you try to address how you feel and to process and deal with it in a positive way. We will show you how you might achieve this. We will also point you in the direction of trained people who can help you if you want or need additional support.

Women

Women are often the first to realize that there may be a fertility problem. As you begin to suspect that having a baby may not be straightforward for you, so your confidence and self-esteem may take a dip, and nagging questions start to trouble you. Each month, waiting to see whether or not your period is going to start can begin to dominate your life. You spend half your month in a state of barely contained expectation and the remainder in a state of upset when a pregnancy doesn't occur. Sound familiar? It's uncomfortable, isn't it?

As we have seen in the previous chapter, at this stage it's natural for you to encounter a wide range of emotions. Perhaps you are astonished and angry that pregnancy hasn't happened easily and spontaneously for you, especially after years spent using contraceptive methods. You may feel responsible in some way and that you are letting your partner down. Or are you wracked with guilt? Do you believe that something you did in the past is causing your present inability to become pregnant? You probably know that it's irrational to believe you're being punished for some previous wrongdoing, but you'd be amazed how many women confess that this is how they feel. You're not alone in thinking this way but let us say in the strongest possible terms, **you should not feel guilty**. You have not done anything to deserve what you are currently going through. Your biggest concern may be how to convince your partner that help and advice, or even medical intervention, is necessary. Does he think you're panicking too soon?

All of the above scenarios are commonplace, albeit this does not make them any less real or upsetting. However, there are strategies to help you to cope with these emotions and to get through this 'Is there or isn't there a problem?' stage that precedes investigations and a definite diagnosis.

> *MYTH: Without medical intervention, a diagnosis of 'infertility' means a lifetime without natural children.*
>
> **FACT:** A diagnosis of unexplained infertility, which is when medical tests and investigations can show no explanation for why you're not getting pregnant, is distressing. Yet, you hear of couples who have had to accept that they are infertile and cannot have children who find, to their astonishment, and sometimes as long as ten years after first trying for a baby, that a pregnancy occurs. It is unusual without medical assistance, but it happens.

Coping strategies

- At this early stage, it is important that you and your partner communicate well. It may not always be easy, but you need to support each other now. Explaining what each of you is feeling is important.

- Be prepared for the fact that your feelings and those of your partner may differ, and that you may be at different stages of concern. You should both remember that each person's viewpoint is valid.

- It is natural to be preoccupied with your fertility issues but it is not good for you to become consumed by them. Try to redirect your focus to positive things such as your favourite hobby or pastime, or why not try a new activity?

- Your feelings of frustration and anger are perfectly natural and expressing them to someone that you trust can be helpful. If you do not want to discuss your fears with friends and family as yet, then consider a telephone helpline or seeing a counsellor.

- Consult your doctor and discuss your concerns with him or her. Although it may be too soon to start investigations (remember, you should allow a year of trying before undergoing tests if you're under 35), you will probably feel a huge sense of relief once you acknowledge that there's a problem and seek help.

Q. Sometimes I feel as though I don't care whether or not I have a baby. It's as if I'm completely numb. Am I abnormal?

A. When emotions are very painful and overwhelming, it is understandable that we sometimes want to take a break from them. The numbness you describe is your way of protecting yourself and it's perfectly normal. It doesn't mean that you don't care or that you don't want a baby – in fact, quite the reverse. It would probably be a good idea to talk to your partner, supportive friends or family members or a trained counsellor to help you express how you are feeling.

Your partner

You know only too well the distressing effect that a delay in getting pregnant is having on you, but it is also important to recognize your partner's feelings and the damage that repeated disappointment can have on your relationships in general, but especially with him.

MYTH: Men are less upset by infertility than women.

FACT: Cultural conditioning dictates that men often show their emotions less than women. You know the score: big boys don't cry, take it like a man, etc. But, even if they don't show or discuss how they are feeling, don't make the mistake of thinking that men who are facing fertility problems are not experiencing the same upsetting and maddening emotions that women are.

Women often have a support network of good friends and family with whom they can unburden. This is not always the case with men who often benefit a great deal from talking to a counsellor about their emotions and what they are experiencing, assuming you can convince them to seek help.

At this time, both of you need a great deal of loving support, patience and reassurance. Try to talk openly to one another about how you are feeling. Remember that what causes you most pain may not be the same for him, and vice versa.

Perhaps he is upset that the spontaneity of lovemaking has gone and that the pure joy of physical intimacy and sex is now ruined. Or does he secretly wonder if you now want a baby more than you want him? Would your partner prefer to enlist the support of friends and relatives while you prefer not to tell anyone just yet? If each of you can discuss your opinions and express your own fears as candidly as possible, you will be able to help each other more easily.

If you get to the stage where an investigation of your fertility situation is called for, then you may be asked to make a decision on whether or not you want medical assistance or intervention. This is a deeply personal choice and it's a decision that, as a couple, you should try to take together (treatment options and cost implications are discussed in Chapter 4). The good news is that if you are already accustomed to talking to each other openly about your feelings and emotions, hard decisions such as these will be clearer and, dare we say, hopefully easier to make.

In some cases, facing the shared anguish of delayed conception and infertility can make you closer. Some couples, especially those who keep their inability to have children a secret, report that they experienced a kind of 'us against the world' feeling, and that being united in overcoming their problem made the relationship stronger. Whatever the final outcome, whether you have a child together, with help or by adoption, or whether you choose to lead a fulfilling life without children, you may have a more united, loving relationship as a result of your experiences.

Nonetheless, a delay in getting pregnant is an emotional and physical hurdle for both of you – and sometimes it is a lot to face on your own, so why not consider calling upon friends and relatives to lend their emotional support?

Irrespective of whether you deal with the early stages of delayed conception as a couple or involve other people, you can still make it your priority to enjoy one another's company and to give each other support, love and reassurance. After all, a good relationship is a great gift. It's hard, we know, but you must both try to live in the present, not the future.

How can you relieve the emotional stress?

We all have busy lives and we are all vulnerable to stress, but couples suffering from infertility find themselves caught in a vicious circle. Are you infertile because you are stressed, or are you stressed because you are infertile? Of course, it is more complex than that, but what is certain is that too much stress can adversely affect your chances of getting pregnant. Studies show that a man's sperm production decreases in response to stress and there are a few studies that show that the failure of women to menstruate during wartime may be just one example of the detrimental effect that emotions have on fertility.

At this point, it's worth acknowledging that although stress can be damaging when you're trying to get pregnant, if there is a physical reason for your failure to conceive, well-meaning people telling you to 'relax and it will happen' are not only irritating but downright unhelpful. We sympathize with you if you hear this all too often, but please remember that although reducing stress may not always be the answer to your problems, it can help you to cope with the strain of infertility a little better. Let's look at what you can do to reduce your stress levels.

Q. When I see mothers in the street ignoring their children, I feel so full of resentment. Why have they got children that they don't seem to want when I can't have the child that I would dearly love?

A. Many couples experiencing delayed conception or infertility confess to feeling very bitter when they witness what appears to be neglect or disinterest. It's like having salt rubbed in the wound, and yours is a perfectly understandable reaction. Yet, ultimately, resentment and bitterness will only harm you and your chances of conceiving. You have taken the first positive step in acknowledging these feelings, but it may be helpful to work through your reactions in more depth with a qualified therapist or counsellor who will help you to see how bitterness can impact on other areas of your life.

What you can do

If you and your partner think that stress might be getting to you, look for ways to minimize its effects in your life. Not all of the following ideas will appeal to you, and don't adopt any of these suggestions because you feel 'you ought to' – that will simply make you more stressed. However, some of these options might suit you.

- **Physical exercise counteracts stress.** Try to build more activity into your life, even if it is only walking to the shop to pick up the newspaper. If you can do some exercise, such as swimming, dancing or yoga, for example, so much the better.

- **Learn to say no.** Taking on too much can be very stressful. A firm but polite refusal will not be taken the wrong way.

- **Bring some levity into your life.** Give yourself a chance to laugh more by watching comedies, reading light humorous novels and mixing with good friends.

- **Join a relaxation class or listen to relaxation tapes at home.** These are especially beneficial at night if you have difficulty sleeping.

- **Indulge in your hobbies more often.** Whether it is dancing or painting, an activity that you find fulfilling and absorbing will be relaxing.

- **A massage is a great way to relieve the physical tensions induced by stress.** If you don't fancy stripping off, perhaps a reflexology treatment (foot massage) or head massage would be best.

- **Remember to control your breathing.** Use the exercise that we suggest in Chapter 1 (page 12), or simply focus on your breathing and make sure you breathe slowly and from the abdomen, not just into the top of your lungs.

- **Limit your working hours.** You know what they say about all work and no play! But, more seriously, working long hours puts an undue strain on you.

If your stress levels remain high despite trying some of the above techniques, then you can consult your doctor who might refer you to a counsellor or a psychotherapist.

On the spot stress buster

If you find yourself in an uncomfortable situation and you can feel your anxiety levels rising, just try the following coping strategy to get you through the difficult moment. At first, practice the procedure at home in a quiet, safe environment. Once mastered, you can employ it at any time and anywhere.

- Sit comfortably and close your eyes (this won't be necessary once you've got the hang of it!).
- Imagine a scene that represents for you peace and tranquillity. A safe haven if you like. It might be on a beach, in a secluded garden or high on a mountain. It can be a real place or somewhere in your imagination. The most important thing is that you find it quiet and relaxing.
- Picture yourself in your private place and exclude everything else around you.
- If you have time, you can also visualize

the situation that you wish for, perhaps you're pregnant or maybe you have your baby, and allow your mind the freedom to explore.

• When you've finished, open your eyes and be amazed at how the stress has just drained away.

Note: This is an example of visualization, a technique that is used by sportspeople, practitioners and counsellors to boost positive feelings, reduce anxiety, improve self-image and strengthen emotional and mental health. You can find out more from a practitioner – see Part 5, Chapter 12.

Dealing with other people

When you're desperately hoping to get pregnant, the most dreaded question in any social gathering is 'Do you have children?' We know how wretched you feel when these questions arise but, unfortunately, they are not going to go away. Painful and uncomfortable though it may be for you, it is best to give some prior thought to how you might answer such enquiries. We recommend that you keep your answer short and to the point – you don't have to explain yourself – and then steer the conversation to safer ground.

Even without having to deal with pointed questions, it is easy and understandable to find yourself feeling angry at the sight of a young mother pushing a pram with a toddler by her side. Why her and not me, you ask yourself. These self-doubts and painful reactions are completely natural, yet you cannot and should not shut yourself away from a world that is full of painful reminders. Don't forget, it may be you pushing the pram in the near future.

However, we understand that it is natural to want to protect yourself from distressing reminders – and we certainly don't advocate putting yourself in uncomfortable positions if you have a choice. Avoid playgrounds in parks, for example, and don't agree to attend antenatal classes with a friend who's going to be a single mum: that's just too much to expect of yourself.

It's not a good idea to try to hide from everyday life either. It only makes you feel more isolated and lonely. Instead, why not try to throw yourself into the things that you and your partner love to do and try to embrace the life you already have together? Easy for us to say, you're probably thinking, and that's true. It would be glib to pretend that this strategy is easy, but it's worth a try if you can manage it.

We want to assure you that you are not alone with your problem and you may find that through talking with others in a similar situation, you feel reassured and much better. If you don't know anyone who is also having delays or difficulty in starting a family, then a support group such as those run by the Infertility Network UK (see Part 5 for details) may be just what you need.

Involving friends and relatives

It is hard to know at what stage to tell your friends and family that you are having problems with conception. Many couples prefer not to mention their difficulties until they have exhausted the time in which they might reasonably hope to get pregnant naturally, and they are well on the path to investigations and possible treatment.

Depending on the closeness of your relationships, you might prefer to involve parents, relatives and friends at an earlier stage. Once again, this is a highly personal decision and you will probably find, as you discuss the matter with your partner, that there are pros and cons to both options. For example, if you keep the fact that you're having difficulty getting pregnant to yourselves, then you'll probably have to field innocent but tactless questions such as, 'When are you going to start a family?' and 'What are you waiting for?' Or even worse, 'Don't you want children?'

Have you noticed how relations and close friends seem to feel that their blood ties and familiarity give them the right to ask over-bold and intrusive questions? Yet they don't mean to hurt you. Like most people, they simply haven't considered that you might be having difficulties.

Alternatively, if you tell trusted family and friends about your problems, they may be a source of great support, or they could be at a loss as to what to say. Even people who know you exceptionally well and who wish to be supportive may struggle to find the right words and to offer the right comfort. Some friends, especially those with young children or who are expecting a child, might even avoid you rather than cause an uncomfortable situation. This can be extremely hurtful but they are doing it because they don't want to make things worse for you.

You're the best judge of how your loved ones might react, how helpful they may be and whether or not you can discuss their discomfort and tell them how best to behave around you. If it's too uncomfortable to discuss openly, you can always show them the guide for relatives and friends section in this chapter (page 50), or simply photocopy it and leave it for them to read. Try to bear in mind that your loved ones will not consciously mean to cause you pain. They simply do not know how to act for the best.

Finding a natural listener

It's an unfortunate fact of life that some people will say the wrong things, and some people are incredibly crass and insensitive in difficult situations, but others will say the right things and will be a great source of support and comfort for you. Some people might say very little at all and just be natural and relaxed around you, as they have always been. This in itself can be reassuring at a time when life seems anything but natural.

You will almost certainly have someone in your group of friends and relatives – perhaps a girlfriend or maybe your mother – who is naturally good at listening without judgement, and being with them is not only hugely supportive, but such a relief. Rest assured, there's someone that you know and trust who will be there for you and who will be able to make you feel good. This is an important point. At this challenging time, you should seek out the company of people who make you feel comfortable, relaxed and good about yourself; basically, the friends and relatives who enrich your life. By the same token, there are always people in our circle of friends and family who are demanding and draining – and you should give these people a wide berth at the moment. This is not being selfish – it's important to be kind to yourself and to avoid any unnecessary hassle until you find yourself in a less stressful period of your life.

Q. My friend went to see a counsellor when she was suffering from depression after her divorce. She thought she was excellent and has recommended her to me. I'd prefer to follow my friend's personal recommendation but do I need to see someone who specializes in infertility issues?

A. A counsellor is trained to help you process the destructive effect of the emotions you are experiencing, and in many ways the cause of your anger or frustration, etc. is immaterial. If you get to the stage where you and your partner decide to undergo assisted conception, then good clinics very often have in-house counsellors whose expertise obviously lies in this area. However, in the initial stages of delayed conception, your friend's recommendation is probably a good one to follow.

Getting additional help

We know what a strain you are under, and facing your feelings is not always easy to do on your own. You deserve some emotional and psychological support and, if you can't find someone in your circle of friends and professional carers – consider your partner, your best friend, your mum or sister, your doctor or complementary practitioner – then it can be a good idea to go to a counsellor or therapist for help in coping with and processing your emotions.

Why not ask your doctor to refer you to a therapist trained in dealing with the stress of infertility at all stages of its management? Don't worry – everything you say to a counsellor is heard in confidence. Irrespective of how swamped by your emotions you have felt before and during a session, at the end of your appointment you should feel confident about going back out into the world and facing people again.

It may also be useful to attend sessions as a couple. In many instances, partners say things in the presence of a counsellor that they wouldn't otherwise disclose, and this can be illuminating for you both.

Occasionally, counselling is available on the UK's National Health Service (NHS) but, more often, you have to pay privately, with sessions costing in the region of £30-£50 per hour. It's vital to make sure that any counsellor you go to is fully qualified and registered with a professional body. If your doctor does not refer you, then the British Association for Counselling and Psychotherapy (see Part 5, Chapter 12 for details) has a list of local practitioners.

A guide for relatives and friends

When someone you care about opens up to you and tells you that they are having problems conceiving a child, they are likely to be feeling upset and extremely sensitive to any comments you might make. Although you may not know what to say for the best, a caring and supportive attitude from you can make all the difference to how they're able to deal with their problem.

Couples who have been through the painful experience of fertility problems report that the following approaches from concerned loved ones are the most helpful.

- It's preferable that you show an interest in their problems and ask how things are going (or ask if it's okay to ask) rather than saying nothing because you don't want to upset them (which can give the impression that you don't care).

- Although you mean well, giving advice such as 'It's only a matter of time' or 'Don't try too hard' and other such homilies only serves to make the couple feel inadequate and as if it's their fault (which it isn't). It's probably best to leave the advice to the experts.

- Offering reassurance and encouragement is good but holding out unrealistic promises of definite success is not helpful.

- You can be sympathetic. Offering a sympathetic listening ear is probably the most supportive thing you can do.

- Don't try to jolly them along. Infertility can be a devastating experience and telling them that things could be worse or that kids only mess up your home only serves to trivialize their problems rather than cheer them up.

- You cannot protect the couple from other people's pregnancies. It is often better for the couple to hear about a new pregnancy from you without delay, so they can get used to the idea. Surprise pregnancy announcements in public can be upsetting and so it's kinder to let them know beforehand. Some couples appreciate it if a friend tells them they are planning a pregnancy too.

- Infertility often feels like a failure by the couples affected and it erodes self-esteem. Some only confide their problems to close family and friends while others prefer it if everyone knows so that they don't put their foot in it. It's best to respect the couple's wishes.

- Making jokes about infertility or using derogatory terms for infertile men and women is unlikely to produce a laugh. Be sensitive to the situation. Occasionally, couples can joke about their own plight but you should never initiate the joking.

Coming from an Asian background, infertility is something that is not discussed openly although we ourselves didn't feel that there was a stigma. We told a few people outside our immediate family and friends and I distanced myself from some people who I felt were not supportive for a while.

We felt it was quite personal and didn't want everyone knowing. We didn't want to keep telling everyone if cycles failed at a time when we were still trying to get our own heads around it.

People think that because they got pregnant easily, it's easy for everyone and they can come out with hurtful comments. Although unintentional, you are very vulnerable when you are going through treatment.

Seeta

I found facing the reality of not being able to conceive was the hardest thing I have ever had to do in my life. But there is excellent support out there for couples like us. We learned so much about ourselves, our bodies and each other and we take nothing for granted now. It has been difficult – almost impossible sometimes – but we are closer, more appreciative of each other, and healthier than ever before.

Amy

I was totally obsessed with trying to become pregnant. The thoughts were with me 24 hours a day and affected everything I did. I wouldn't even buy new clothes for myself because I was sure that I would soon be pregnant and would need maternity clothes. I didn't expect to have so much trouble, and instead of taking each day at a time, I just obsessed about getting pregnant to the exclusion of everything else.

Sarah

Part 2:
Taking Action –
Practical Steps

3

Moving forward

In Part 1, we looked specifically at your probable first reactions to finding out that getting pregnant might not be straightforward for you, and how this discovery might make you feel. Now in Part 2 we concentrate on helping you to decide what steps to take next.

You are on the verge of making your first moves towards your chosen outcome. In other words, you are taking positive action to help you get pregnant, and that often brings with it a sense of relief and perhaps some sense of regaining control in your life. Our focus in this chapter is on arming you with the knowledge to make choices. Initially, this probably means getting confirmation from your doctor of your current fertility position and the options available. From here, you can decide how *you* want to handle the situation and how *you* want to proceed towards your goal of having a baby.

We'll explain what we know about the reasons for infertility and then, with a better understanding of the possible causes that may be affecting you, in Chapter 4, we explore and try to make sense of the various treatments that are on offer. These range from self-help measures, such as making changes to your diet and lifestyle, through complementary treatments to drug and medical assistance. In fact, there is such a diverse range of possibilities that one or more of these approaches is bound to suit you and your partner. With so many options to choose from, the chances of having a baby after difficulties in conceiving are better now than they have ever been.

As well as advice on the practical steps you can take, we outline in Chapter 5 the emotional reactions you might expect as you go through various treatments (if that's what you decide), and give you lots of suggestions on how to help yourself and where to get emotional support, including from other women experiencing infertility problems. For now, let's get started on taking the situation into your own hands by looking at how to seek advice and how to get a diagnosis.

Consulting your doctor

The first step in moving forward is a visit to your doctor and, if at all possible, you should go with your partner. We recommend this because you are both going to have to undergo some simple tests in order to find out the reason, if any, for your problems, so it's useful if your partner is involved from the outset.

Your doctor will listen to your concerns and make a note of your medical history. Don't worry – your doctor will be sympathetic and will take your fears seriously, irrespective of how long you've been trying. He or she may give you a physical examination followed by a few basic tests or you may be invited to make another appointment for the tests.

These initial investigations, called primary tests in medical jargon, will probably consist of:

- **Blood tests**. You will be asked to give a blood sample seven days before your period is due to see if you are ovulating, and another during your period to check for any hormone imbalances. They will also check your blood for immunity to German measles (rubella) because if you contract this disease during the first three months of a pregnancy, it can harm your unborn baby.

- If you haven't had a **cervical smear test** recently, that will probably be organized too.

- Both you and your partner may have a **urine test** to check for chlamydia, which is a sexually transmitted disease (see page 69) that can result in damaged fallopian tubes in women and damaged ejaculatory ducts in men, preventing you from becoming pregnant.

- Your partner will be asked to give a **sperm sample** to check for abnormalities.

MYTH: A doctor only has seven minutes in which to treat a patient.

FACT: Doctor's waiting rooms are notoriously crowded and it is true that, on average, each patient sees a doctor for less than ten minutes. However, exceptions can always be made. If you explain the nature of your appointment in advance, the receptionist can arrange a full half hour's appointment for you, probably at a less pressurized time of day, so that you can have a more detailed and relaxed conversation with your doctor. Before your appointment it is worth making some time to note down anything that you think your doctor should know about so that you avoid wasting time.

MYTH: Masturbation is bad for male fertility.

FACT: A man does not have a finite number of sperm that could run out – the testicles produce and store sperm from puberty throughout adult life, and masturbation does not damage sperm quality or quantity.

Sperm count jargon buster

The primary analysis of your partner's semen sample is to establish his sperm count. This is then classified by the following medical terms, which may sound disconcerting but don't be put off. They are actually pretty clear-cut once you become accustomed to the strange-sounding names:

- **Azoospermia**. There are no sperm in the semen, either as a result of a blockage affecting the movement of the sperm, failure to ejaculate or inability to make sperm.

- **Oligospermia**. More widely known as a low sperm count, there are some sperm present but not as many as normal. In fact, less than 20 million sperm per millilitres of semen is classified as oligospermia. (Believe it or not, as many as 300 million sperm in total can be released on ejaculation.)

- **Aesthenospermia**. The sperm are unable to wriggle and move as they should. This is known as low motility, even if the sperm count is normal.

- **Teratospermia**. The semen contains a high number of abnormal sperm (sperm with split heads, no tails and other abnormalities).

- **Aspermia**. There is no ejaculation.

So what's normal?

In a semen sample, a healthy analysis should contain:

- over 20 million sperm per millilitre

- more than half the sperm wriggling (motility)

- more than one-third normal sperm

- a normal white blood cell count (less than 1 million per millilitre of sperm).

What comes next?

If your primary test results are normal and you have been trying for a baby for less than 12 months (six months if you're over 35), then your doctor may offer some self-help suggestions (see Chapter 4, page 95) for maximizing your fertility, but they will probably suggest that you try for a little longer before referring you for further investigations.

Having taken the first step of going to see your doctor, it's only natural to feel disappointed at being told to wait a bit longer, but try to be consoled by the fact that your tests were normal. You stand a very good chance of getting pregnant on your own – it may just take longer than you might have hoped.

However, your doctor will probably refer you for further, more detailed tests (termed 'secondary tests' in the medical professions) if:

- Your primary tests reveal a possible fertility issue

- Your physical examinations show any abnormality in the shape of your pelvic/genital anatomy or your partner has a varicocoele on his scrotum (see glossary)

- Your monthly menstrual cycle is less than 21 days or more than 35 days

- You have a previous medical history of gynaecological conditions such as pelvic inflammatory disease (PID), an ectopic pregnancy or endometriosis

- If you have been trying for a baby for one year or more (12– 18 months if you are in your early thirties and more than six months if you're over 35).

Q. What is an ovulation prediction kit and why would I want one?

A. These kits offer a fairly sophisticated way of plotting your ovulation cycle so that you can ensure you are having intercourse at the best time to conceive. They are widely available at chemists and there are even a few supermarkets that stock them. You use a urine dipstick to monitor your hormone levels and to find out when you are about to ovulate. Although they can be helpful, they are not strictly accurate and can give misleading readings. They are also pretty expensive so you may not want to rely on using them for any length of time.

MYTH: If you have no symptoms, you don't have a sexually transmitted disease (STD).

FACT: One of the most common STDs, chlamydia, is a microscopic parasite and many people who have been infected are quite unaware that they have the disease. In fact, up to 70 per cent of women with chlamydia have no symptoms. The problem is that chlamydia can cause pelvic inflammatory disease (PID), and one incidence of PID has a 10 per cent chance of causing tubal blockage (a common cause of infertility), with the risk rising to 50 per cent after three episodes. It is very important to check for chlamydia infection as part of your primary investigations.

MYTH: A small penis makes less sperm.

FACT: There is no correlation between the size of the penis and the quality or quantity of sperm produced. A man with a small penis could produce more sperm in quality and quantity than a man with a large penis. It bears no relation.

Sex lives suffering from pressure?

Sometimes, the demand to have sex at the appropriate time becomes yet another pressure and can turn what used to be playful, loving and fun into a chore. Occasionally, the strain to perform becomes so great that, for men, it becomes difficult to get or sustain an erection or to ejaculate. For women, intercourse can become painful as a lack of arousal results in vaginal dryness or muscle tension.

If you find that you and your partner are no longer enjoying your love life and that you have distracting thoughts during sex about whether this time will be *the* time, then it's probably a good idea to look at new ways to bring some renewed intimacy and energy back into your sex life. Why not try some of the following suggestions?

- Vary your sex life. Have sex around the time of ovulation by all means but also enjoy having sex at other times.

- Avoid planned sex, especially if one of you does not feel in the mood at the appointed time.

- Make time for each other and do things, as a couple, that does not have baby-making as its focus. How about a trip away or days out together?

- Remember to keep talking and to keep telling each other that you care – invest in each other.

If the problems with your love life persist, then Relate, the UK relationship counselling charity (see Part 5, Chapter 12), has trained sex therapists who are sure to be able to help.

Q. My partner and I have just seen our doctor for the first time because we've been trying for a baby for 15 months and nothing has happened. He asked about the kind of work we do. What has our occupation got to do with having a baby?

A. Some occupations involve dangers that can adversely affect fertility, especially for men, who are particularly vulnerable to certain hazards that can depress their sperm count. For example, working with pesticides, X-rays, solvents such as those used in photocopiers and paint products, and heavy metals such as lead, mercury or arsenic. High temperatures are known to damage sperm production so if your husband is a factory worker or a baker, for instance, this may have some bearing on the situation.

It may or may not have been relevant in your case, but workplace hazards can be a contributory cause of infertility that can be easily identified and rectified for some couples, which is why your doctor was asking.

Secondary tests

The next step in finding out why you're not getting pregnant is to undergo more specialized investigations called 'secondary tests'. Your doctor will refer you to your local hospital or fertility clinic for these.

The tests can sound daunting and you may be a little anxious about attending a specialist clinic but you really shouldn't be worried. Specialist infertility clinics are staffed by professional, multi-skilled teams who will help you through the investigations in a friendly, relaxed and sympathetic way. Rest assured that they really want to provide the best outcome for you both, namely a healthy baby, and they will do everything in their power to make the experience as comfortable as possible for you. The clinic staff will explain carefully and in detail the nature of the tests that you and your partner will undergo, but for now, here is a brief preview of what you and your partner might expect.

Secondary tests for women

If your primary tests indicate that you are ovulating, then there's a range of more detailed investigations available to help discover why you have not been able to conceive as yet.

- **Ultrasound scan:** To check your womb and ovaries and to confirm that you're ovulating.

- **Follicle tracking:** By ultrasound, to follow the development of a follicle and tracking it to see if an egg is developing.

- **Endometrial biopsy:** A tissue sample is taken from your womb's lining to be analysed for a normal microscopic appearance, but this test is not common. If offered, the sample will be taken during the second half of your menstrual cycle when any changes in the endometrial lining due to progesterone levels will be visible.

- **HyCoSy (hysterocontrastsalpingography):** The fallopian tubes and uterine cavity are assessed using a transvaginal ultrasound that looks at the passage of dye from the uterine cavity along the fallopian tubes and to the ovaries.

- **Hysterosalpingogram (HSG):** Dye is injected into the cavity of the uterus and fallopian tubes, and an X-ray is then taken to check for blockages in your fallopian tubes.

- **Laparoscopy:** A dye is injected through your cervix and a fibre-optic camera is then inserted through the abdominal wall to enable the surgeon to view your internal organs and to check for tubal blockages.

- **Hysteroscopy:** Similar to a laparoscopy. A specialized endoscope (flexible telescope) is used to view your uterus to check for conditions such as adhesions (scar tissue), fibroids and other problems.

All of the above tests are quite intimate and intrusive in nature, but the trained staff will try to make you feel as relaxed and comfortable as possible. If you can, be comforted by the fact that they are seeing and helping women just like you on a daily basis, so there is no need to feel embarrassed.

Q. I didn't have any trouble getting pregnant with my son, so why is it taking so long this time?

A. Whether or not you had your son with your current partner or with a previous partner, you can still find it difficult to conceive a second or subsequent time. In fact, secondary infertility (as your situation is called) affects about 5 per cent of the UK population.

Could there have been changes in your lifestyle that could be influencing your fertility as a couple? For example, have you or your partner had any medical problems? Are you more stressed at work? Do you have sex as frequently as you did when you were last trying for a baby? Your age is also a factor and you may not be quite as fertile as you were if you've left it some years to have a second child. It is worth consulting your doctor to investigate some of these and other possible causes.

We realize how frustrating it must be to experience delays in conception after having no problems the first time but try not to worry too much. It may be a change in your lifestyle that's the cause, and this can be easily rectified, or it may simply be the case that it will take longer to happen this time around.

Feeling the strain

The wait for test results can be quite lengthy and this is a stressful time for both you and your partner. To take your mind off the wait, try to make time for each other and do the things you love. Remind yourselves that you are doing all that you can at the moment and there is no sense in worrying too much about the things that you can't control. If possible, keep following the self-help lifestyle changes in Chapter 4 – eating healthily, taking time to relax, enjoying your sex life and spending time with each other, and remember, **you're moving forward**.

Secondary tests for men

Over the past 50 years, sperm counts in the developed world have declined, and some scientists believe this may be due in part to environmental causes (see Chapter 4, page 101). Nonetheless, with advances in investigation procedures and in treatments, there's a greater chance than ever before that men with sub-fertility issues can be helped to achieve natural fatherhood.

Sometimes the biggest hurdle to treatment can be getting men to accept help because, sadly, many men still equate fertility with virility. We all know that this is not the case – a man with a low sperm count can be a fantastic lover, just as the opposite may be true, but your partner may need a little reassurance and support on the subject. Knowing what to expect can help and he may be reassured to know that the tests for men are non-invasive and pretty straightforward.

Semen analysis

After routine semen analysis at the primary test stage to check a man's sperm count, microscopic inspection of his semen samples at the secondary stage of investigation may be carried out to examine the:

- sperm's ability to recognize the ovum (egg) and latch on to it (acrosome test)

- sperm's ability to swim through the cervical mucus and reach the uterus (sperm invasion test)

- sperm's ability to fuse with and fertilize the ovum (egg penetration test)

- presence of protein molecules that may prevent sperm fertilizing an ovum (sperm antibody test). Note: This test is very rarely performed, and usually only in a research setting.

Your partner will be asked to give at least two semen samples for analysis because sperm counts vary from day to day and even hour to hour (it's affected by all sorts of things such as illness, medication and how often you have sex.)

Q. My partner has problems getting an erection. Can this be treated? I'm worried that it's damaging our chances of having a baby.

A. In about 5 per cent of couples, a problem with sex is the principal cause of infertility. Impotence, an inability to attain or maintain an erection firm enough for intercourse, can be caused by physical reasons such as diabetes or diseases of the nervous system and your partner should be reassured that these causes can be treated. However, in many cases, the underlying cause of impotence is psychological and the pressure inherent in trying for a baby can aggravate the situation. Again, let your partner know that counselling can be a great help in treating this problem.

Why are you unable to conceive?

There is rarely a single cause for infertility, and getting through all the tests can be a lengthy and frustrating process. We know it's not always easy to be patient, but try to bear in mind that by taking the time to eliminate various causes, the doctors stand a better chance of finding a treatment that will work for you.

Possible problems for women

It is possible that, after investigation, you will still have no explanation for your difficulties in getting pregnant. However, there are some common and generally treatable reasons for infertility that may be identified by tests. These include the following:

Hormonal imbalances

Problems caused by abnormal levels of hormones, such as a failure to ovulate, are the most common reasons for female infertility and are found in about one-third of all infertile women. For 90 per cent of these women, drug treatments will rectify the imbalance and restore regular ovulation.

Polycystic ovaries

Polycystic ovary syndrome (PCOS) is a common condition that affects as many as one in five women during their reproductive years. Polycystic means that the ovaries contain a number of small fluid-filled sacks (cysts), each about 4 mm across. The cause of polycystic ovaries is unknown, and in the majority of women, it only leads to minor problems associated with their periods. However, for some of these women, there is a variety of hormonal problems, including infertility.

Polycystic ovaries can be treated. In some women, a surgical procedure can be performed called 'ovarian drilling'. Using a laparoscope and a hot probe, the surgeon will puncture the ovarian tissue in up to five points. We do not know how the treatment works but it can be enough to start you ovulating regularly, so restoring fertility. For others, the treatment involves taking a drug at the beginning of the cycle to stimulate ovulation and this can be enough to help you to become pregnant. In more extreme cases (which are quite rare we should point out), injections of hormones may be needed to re-establish fertility (administered at a specialist infertility unit).

Endometriosis

This is a condition where fragments from the lining of the womb (the endometrium) become attached to sites outside the womb, principally on the ovaries, the peritoneum (the thin lining that covers all the organs of the abdomen), the fallopian tubes, the cervix, in the vagina, or the ligaments around the womb, uterus and bladder. As the endometrium grows during your menstrual cycle, so too do the fragments, often causing severe pain.

Opinion is divided on how common endometriosis is, but it would seem that about 10–15 per cent of women may suffer from the disease and, unfortunately, it can cause difficulties in becoming pregnant. Once diagnosed (usually by laparoscopy), there are two main forms of treatment:

- drug therapy with hormones

- laser surgery.

Both are supervised and administered at a specialist infertility clinic.

Tubal blockage

One-third of all cases of female infertility are as a result of a tubal blockage. The most common cause of blocked tubes is infection, and the most common infection implicated is chlamydia (see page 69). In fact, as many as 70 per cent of women who have blocked tubes have had a chlamydia infection, although most of the time they weren't even aware they'd had it.

Tubal blockages can only be detected at the secondary test stage of investigation. However, the good news is that, in some cases, it is possible to have surgery to open the blocked tubes, or occasionally a small section of blocked tube can be removed, so raising the chances of you getting pregnant.

Ectopic pregnancy

Sad to say, the delight of becoming pregnant is very occasionally short-lived when a pregnancy develops in the fallopian tubes instead of the uterus. This is known as an ectopic pregnancy and the cause is unknown.

Once an ectopic pregnancy is confirmed, an operation must be carried out to remove the pregnancy and, sometimes, part of the fallopian tube or even part of the ovary too. Unfortunately, this treatment can sometimes cause tubal damage, leading to infertility. An ectopic pregnancy is naturally very distressing, but many women who have had an ectopic pregnancy go on to enjoy a normal pregnancy and delivery.

Lifestyle hazards

In Chapter 4, we discuss some basic lifestyle changes that you can make to optimize your chances of conceiving but, for now, let's take a look at some lifestyle hazards that may be damaging your chances of conceiving.

- **Stress** can lead to anovulation (failure to ovulate) in women and to a reduced sperm count in men.

- **Vigorous physical workouts** can contribute to infertility and, conversely, a complete lack of exercise is also a factor. Why not replace strenuous workouts with something a little less demanding? And, if you're a beginner, try yoga, Tai chi and other gentle exercise regimes, including walking.

- **Poor nutrition.** Both you and your partner should eat a balanced diet rich in fruits and vegetables and low in processed foods (which contain additives and preservatives) whenever possible.

- **Smoking, drinking and street drugs.** These habits can damage the sperm and ova (eggs), and pose a threat to your future baby.

- **Contraception.** In particular, women who have been on the contraceptive pill or used the copper IUD (interuterine device) can experience fertility issues.

- **Environmental oestrogen disruptors.** The environment is polluted with xenoestrogens from pesticides, phthalates (found in nail polish and PVC products), parabens (in cosmetics) and even HRT (hormone replacement therapy) residues in our drinking water.

- **Overweight or underweight.** Either end of the spectrum can compromise your chances of conceiving.

- **Tight fitting clothing.** Loose clothing is better for the body when you're trying for a baby.

- **Lack of sex.** Sounds obvious, doesn't it, but most fertility clinics recommend the ideal frequency of sexual intercourse for couples trying to conceive is every two to three days.

If one or more of the above categories apply to you or your partner, perhaps you should think about trying to alter a few things in your life. And don't worry, it's never too late to make changes.

Possible problems for men

Historically, infertility was considered solely to be a woman's problem, but since the late 1990s, huge advances have been made in our understanding of male infertility and its treatment. Here are some of the findings and most common causes.

Sperm abnormality

The most common cause of male infertility is a physical problem with the sperm themselves, which are extremely vulnerable. However, even with problems such as low sperm counts and poor motility (see box, page 65–6), it is still possible to conceive normally.

Testicular failure

The cause is often hard to establish but could be due to a chromosomal problem, a blow to the testes (for example, a sports injury), mumps in adulthood or if the testes did not descend properly.

Hormone disorders

This is an unusual cause of infertility in men, but if a problem with the signal from the brain (gonadotrophin deficiency) is identified, then it is usually treatable.

Immunological problems

Occasionally, men produce antibodies that are attached to the sperm, and these can interfere with fertilization by immobilizing or even destroying the sperm. But, take heart – the presence of antibodies does not necessarily put an end to your chances of conceiving.

Helping your sperm count

Men who smoke have a 13–17 per cent lower sperm count than those who do not, and high alcohol intake is also known to markedly reduce sperm count and motility. In addition, tight clothing and prolonged periods of sitting can overheat the testes, causing a reduction in sperm count.

So, if your partner has an abnormal semen analysis, if at all possible, he should try to give up smoking and drinking (over the recommended levels), and he should choose loose fitting trousers and underwear such as boxer shorts.

Cannabis, cocaine and anabolic steroids all have extremely detrimental effects on sperm count, motility and number of normal sperm, so he should avoid these drugs.

Recent research from the US also shows that in over 50 per cent of the men with fertility problems sampled sperm counts soared by 491 per cent after they stopped having baths or using the Jacuzzi and hot tub for a few months. Perhaps swapping to a shower rather than a hot bath could be added to the list of ways your partner can help his sperm count.

When no cause can be found

Even after investigation, sometimes the experts cannot give you a reason for why you are unable to conceive. Although there may be nothing apparently wrong with either you or your partner's reproductive system, you remain without a pregnancy.

This is hard news to hear, we know, but you are not alone and there is still a chance of getting pregnant without intervention. About one in five couples undergoing infertility investigations will be given a diagnosis of unexplained infertility, yet anywhere from 20 per cent to 50 per cent of these couples will eventually conceive, with or without medical assistance.

Going forward

We realize that this is a lot of information to take in all at once and you'll probably want to give yourself time to digest all that we've just discussed, perhaps revisiting the pages that are of most interest to you. That's fine. In fact, it's a good idea to make sure you fully grasp the probable investigations you will undergo if you decide to seek help in having a baby before we move on to the next part on treatments.

When you're worried about your ability to have a baby, it's very important that you have a sense of control and purpose. So, whether you choose to go to your doctor to initiate investigations or whether your plan is to do nothing other than continue to have regular sex for the next six months, it's important from a psychological perspective that you make an active decision. Whatever you choose, it's part of a strategy that you and your partner have agreed. This helps you to feel that you are moving on to the next stage and this sense of purpose is very beneficial.

Of course, we understand that making such far-reaching decisions is not easy, but we hope you will find it reassuring to know that 30–40 per cent of couples who undergo specialist investigation achieve a pregnancy within two years.

After trying for a baby for two years, I was referred for secondary tests and they discovered I had fibroids. Unfortunately, I didn't respond well to drug treatment, so my fertility specialist suggested a myomectomy, which is surgery to remove the fibroids but it leaves the rest of my reproductive organs intact. It's been several months since the operation, and the doctors now tell me that it was a success and to go ahead and try to have a baby because fibroids are no longer an obstacle to getting pregnant.

Sarah

I was only 26 when my periods stopped. At first, I thought I was pregnant, but I was told I'd had an early menopause. I didn't even know that you could have your menopause so early but I now know that about one in every 100 women has a premature menopause, and a few are in their twenties, like me.

I was devastated to find out that I could not have a baby naturally, even though my boyfriend and I hadn't even thought about starting a family at that stage. We were lucky. With the aid of assisted conception, we now have two wonderful children. And I just want other women like me to know that they shouldn't give up hope. It is possible to have a family even after a premature menopause.

Lesley

4

Treatment options

You have taken the first important step of consulting your doctor and undergoing tests for a diagnosis. We hope that having a better understanding of the causes of infertility as discussed in the previous chapter is useful. At the very least, it should help you when it comes to making decisions about how to deal with your particular infertility circumstances.

Unlike an injury, such as a broken leg, or an illness like appendicitis that has only one treatment plan, the causes of delayed conception and infertility tend to be multi-faceted and so the treatment options may be more complex. For some, one approach removes whatever is stopping you from getting pregnant and this is all that's required. However, for others, it helps to think of the treatment options as a pathway: you start with one form of treatment and then, having eliminated that difficulty, you progress to the next until, hopefully, you reach your final goal of a healthy pregnancy and baby. Moreover, remember, there will be help and advice from understanding professionals every step of the way.

What's particularly heartening about seeking help in getting pregnant today is that there are so many different ways to approach the problem, many of which complement each other, so improving success rates still further. For example, you might make lifestyle changes yourself to optimize you and your partner's fertility while having a regular massage to reduce your stress levels, and at the same time, you are undergoing a course of drug treatment from the infertility clinic to boost your ovulation. Each of these different approaches has a place and can be beneficial, and there's almost certainly a treatment option or combination of options that ideally suits you and your specific fertility situation.

Let's take a look at what's on offer and what such treatments might entail. Firstly, we'll look at what you can do to help yourself before going on to explore medical treatments.

Making lifestyle changes

Whether a cause has been found for problems in conceiving or not, did you know that you can give yourself a better chance of becoming pregnant if you are as fit and healthy as you can be? By making some simple changes to your way of life, you are putting yourself in a stronger position to get pregnant. A study conducted in 2001 by the

University of Surrey in England (in conjunction with the charity Foresight) showed that couples with a previous history of infertility who made changes in their lifestyle and diet, and who took nutritional supplements, had an 80 per cent success rate. So, what can you do right now?

Diet

Essential nutrients are needed in your diet if you are going to enjoy the best reproductive health possible. This means eating more fresh produce, fruit and vegetables (organic if possible) and avoiding processed foods, ready-meals and fast foods, if at all possible. Try to vary the foods in your diet and eat a daily helping from the four main food groups – cereals, dairy products, vegetables and fruit, and proteins (meat, fish, nuts and seeds, pulses, milk products, soya products).

Exercise

It is really helpful if you can try to do some physical exercise ideally in the fresh air – three times a week is recommended but every bit helps. Mind you, if you are already a fitness addict, you shouldn't overdo it either – research shows that over-strenuous workouts are as bad for your fertility levels as under-activity. Swimming, walking, dancing, ball sports and cycling are all excellent choices. The Eastern arts of yoga, Pilates, Tai chi and some martial arts are also great if you want to calm the mind as well as work the body.

Sleep

Sleep is often overlooked in our hectic modern lives, but are you getting enough? As you sleep, cell repair and renewal speeds up, blood pressure decreases and stresses are relieved. Good quality regular sleep is essential for a healthy reproductive system.

Alcohol, tobacco and street drugs

We're sure you probably know about the general health risks of smoking, alcohol and street drugs but you may not realize that they can damage the development of sperm and ova (eggs), and be detrimental to your future baby.

We appreciate how hard it can be, but you and your partner should try to give up cigarettes and recreational drugs, or cut down at least, and moderate your alcohol intake while you're trying to conceive. It can be especially hard to do this alone, particularly if your friends and family still partake, so why not consult your doctor who can give you help with giving up or can refer you to the appropriate support network? Alternatively, you could call one of the excellent helplines such as the UK National Health Service (NHS) stop smoking helpline (tel: 0800 169 0169) or the charity Quit (tel: 0800 002 200).

Pollutants

Our environment is heavily polluted and this can negatively affect your fertility. You might think that this is something that's entirely out of your hands, but you can actively lessen the effects of pollutants by buying the best fresh produce, meat and fish you can afford (organic if at all possible) and by filtering your drinking water.

Stress

As discussed earlier, stress can lead to a failure to ovulate in women and a reduced sperm count in men, so if you can reduce your exposure to stressful situations, so much the better. Perhaps you could learn to meditate or join a relaxation class where you will be taught to control your mind and think positively. Your local library may have details of courses in stress management, meditation or relaxation classes.

Watch your weight

If you and your partner can get your weight to the normal bracket for your height, you will greatly improve your chances of getting pregnant since being either over- or underweight can adversely affect fertility. Your doctor can give advice on how to lose weight at a sensible pace since crash diets are not to be recommended at any time, but definitely not when you're trying to conceive when good nutrition is paramount.

Choosing clothing

Men should wear loose fitting underwear that allows circulation of air around the testes, so preventing them from overheating, which can be an obstacle to fertility.

Medication

Certain prescription drugs and over-the-counter drugs can have a detrimental effect on fertility. Make sure you tell your doctor or fertility specialist about any drugs you are taking so a more fertility-friendly alternative can be found.

MYTH: You should only have sex when the woman is ovulating or else the man's sperm will be weakened.

FACT: Making love every day does not produce weakened sperm, and there is nothing to gain by abstaining from sex with the sole aim of producing more vigorous sperm. Most experts recommend that you have penetrative sex about three times a week when trying for a baby, irrespective of where the woman is in her cycle. It is no longer recommended that you confine sex to fertile days only, according to temperature charts or ovulation test kits, because the stress involved in getting the timing right was found to be counterproductive.

Complementary therapies

Complementary therapies as a way to relax you and help you through the stress of undergoing medical intervention can be highly beneficial in supporting conventional treatment.

It is less well known that complementary medicine can also be good for strengthening your general constitution and balancing hormones, so getting your body into optimum health for conception. Some therapies concentrate on the psychological and subconscious factors, which can prevent some couples from conceiving. Of course, this type of therapy cannot help when there is a physical barrier to conception – blocked fallopian tubes, for example, but complementary medicine can be beneficial in helping with unexplained infertility or infertility involving hormone problems and stress. One of the well-known clinics for natural preconceptual care in the UK is Foresight (see Part 5, page 317), and it has helped numerous couples to have a much longed for child.

If you choose to explore the complementary therapies, it is important to make sure you consult a trained and accredited practitioner because many of the herbs and remedies used can have a

Q. I am 37 and my partner is 40. Have we left it too late to have a baby?

A. Not at all! The easiest time for a woman to get pregnant is between the ages of 25 and 38. Admittedly, after that, success rates fall a little but given that couples in their mid-thirties have a seven in ten chance of conceiving within a year, you haven't left it too late at all.

powerful effect on your system. It is also important to tell your doctors that you are using complementary therapies, should you decide to use them alongside conventional infertility treatment. A list of UK governing bodies can be found in Part 5, Chapter 12 (page 311).

As a start though, we offer here a brief overview of some of the therapies that are commonly consulted for infertility and how they might help you:

Acupuncture

This ancient Chinese medical practice involves having fine needles inserted in parts of the body to reduce or increase 'energy' flow, remove blockages, tone and restore balance in the system. It can be successful in treating infertility, particularly when the problem is caused by a lack of periods, problems with ovulation or hormonal deficiency. It is also helpful for older prospective mothers.

Nutritional therapy

Using supplementation with vitamins and minerals together with dietary advice, nutritional therapy can help both you and your partner to improve your overall health, detoxify your body and identify any mineral or vitamin deficiencies.

Herbal medicine

Some herbs have a strong hormonal influence and they have been used over the centuries to promote greater fertility and prevent miscarriage. For men, herbs can boost sperm count and libido.

Many drugs are based on the active elements of plants and you should not underestimate their effects. Although you may have read on websites and in books about certain herbs that can boost fertility etc, we really don't recommend that you self-administer these herbs. Please consult a trained practitioner who can tailor the herbs used and dosages to suit your individual requirements.

Homeopathy

A homeopath will produce an in-depth programme of treatment to suit your specific needs that will cover emotional, hormonal and hereditary symptoms. Remedies can be combined to cover a whole range of possible contributory factors.

Q. We've been trying for a baby for eighteen months. The strain has taken the fun out of our sex life. Is there anything we can do?

A. It is a great shame when the focus of lovemaking becomes about making a baby rather than about fun and expressing your feelings for each other. Making sure that you have a normal sex life throughout the month rather than concentrating on the fertile period can lessen the strain but, if you feel this is affecting your relationship, it could be worth consulting a counsellor who can help you to explore the difficulties you're experiencing as well as working with you to resolve them. The UK organization, Relate (see Part 5) have experienced sex therapists available.

Psychotherapy and counselling

As you saw in Chapter 2, listening therapies can be a source of great support to couples facing problems with fertility. They can offer you ways to help cope with the inevitable stress and emotional tumult that infertility and its treatment can cause. Moreover, if there is an emotional block causing the fertility problem, such as bad experiences in the past, subconscious fears about coping with a pregnancy or childbirth, or worries about the future, counselling or psychotherapy may help you to identify such blocks and resolve them.

Conventional treatment

You may prefer to stick with a more conventional treatment programme, as outlined by your doctor or fertility clinic, in which case there are a number of drug treatments and surgical procedures available that are extremely successful in helping couples to conceive naturally. They are also used to kick-start treatment either before or during in vitro fertilization (IVF).

What drugs would you take?

Ovulation-inducing drugs

For most women who are having ovulation troubles (producing eggs), clomiphene citrate, a hormonal drug usually known simply as Clomid, is prescribed. You will take it in tablet form from the second to the sixth day of your cycle and it works by encouraging the pituitary gland in the brain to produce FSH (follicle-stimulating hormone), a stimulating hormone that makes the ovaries produce eggs. It is advisable to have at least the first cycle of treatment monitored with serial ultrasound scans to make sure only one egg is developing and to avoid having a multiple pregnancy.

Ovulation is monitored by checking your progesterone levels at around day 21 of your cycle. Sometimes, a higher dosage is required and you would then be advised to take two tablets daily for five days (very occasionally it is increased to three tablets daily). You can have up to six cycles of this drug treatment and, encouragingly, over half of women treated become pregnant.

Ovary-stimulating hormones

If Clomid is not successful for you, it may be substituted by FSH injections to stimulate the ovaries over a period of about two weeks. There is a risk of multiple pregnancies with this treatment, but don't worry, you'll be carefully monitored throughout by ultrasound screening. This treatment is particularly useful for women who suffer from polycystic ovary syndrome (PCOS) who have not responded to treatment with Clomid.

Suppressing drugs

If your inability to conceive is caused by high prolactin levels (hyperprolactinaemia), you will probably be given bromocriptine, a drug that suppresses prolactin production and restores ovulation. You will need to take bromocriptine three times a day, but the new generation of similar drugs can be taken once daily or even weekly. These drugs can be highly effective at restoring ovulation and once you become pregnant, treatment then stops.

Drugs such as goserelin and burserelin are cycle-suppressing drugs and are taken as a nasal spray or a daily or monthly injection. They copy the action of natural hormones and are used by doctors to give greater control over your treatment cycle.

Will you need surgery?

If your fallopian tubes are damaged or diseased, perhaps as a result of chlamydia for example, surgery might be the best option for you, particularly if you suffer from pain or other symptoms.

Scarred or narrowed tubes can be unblocked by an operation called tuboplasty, whereby a catheter with a small balloon at the tip is inserted into the blocked tube and the balloon is then gently inflated to allow a way through for the egg. The balloon is then deflated and removed. Alternatively, if the problem lies at the end of the fallopian tube where the ends sometimes becomes fused, a fimbrioplasty operation is used to peel back the end, again allowing the egg to pass. If the delicate internal structure of the tube has been damaged, you will have a higher risk of having a pregnancy in the fallopian tube called an 'ectopic pregnancy' so surgery may not be recommended.

Although in the past, success rates have been disappointing after surgery, these new microsurgical techniques have greatly improved the chances of successfully repairing tubal damage, so improving the likelihood of a healthy pregnancy. However, don't despair if drug treatment or tubal surgery does not work or is not an option for you. You may have exhausted the options for having a baby unassisted, and we understand that this may be upsetting, but there are still a number of highly effective assisted conception techniques that may be suitable for you and your partner and which could help to bring you the baby that you want.

Getting advice

All clinics licensed by the UK's Human Fertilisation and Embryology Authority (HFEA) are obliged to offer you access to what's known as implications counselling before you consent to treatment. This involves a counsellor talking to you about the treatment you plan to have, so that you understand exactly what it involves and how it might affect you and those close to you. Spending time with such a counsellor can help you to adjust to the idea of treatment and to make sure this is the right decision for you.

What is assisted reproduction technology (ART)?

ART is an umbrella term that describes a range of infertility treatments that helps couples to conceive and give birth using the assistance of laboratory techniques. The most well known and common of these treatments is IVF, which literally means 'fertilization in a glass', hence the popular name of 'test-tube' baby. In Britain, around one baby in every 80 is born as a result of IVF treatment. Before we look at IVF in more detail, let's take a moment to discuss intrauterine insemination (IUI), which is a simpler technique and may be the first option for you to consider.

Is ART safe?

None of the procedures used in assisted reproduction technology (ART) should cause any physical danger to you or your partner. They have a remarkably good safety record, and are well regulated and supervised. Some couples are affected psychologically by undergoing assisted conception, and undoubtedly the procedures can be emotionally draining, but you will be offered support and counselling at every step of the journey and there is always someone on hand who can answer your questions, address your concerns and reassure you.

In the UK alone, 6,000 babies a year are born as a result of IVF. It is encouraging to know that so many couples become parents through ART, but we should mention that an assisted conception and pregnancy is at a higher risk than normal of complications, miscarriage or premature birth. Also, multiple pregnancies carry some associated health risks but we can reassure you that your specialist team will be well aware of these medical risks and they'll take great care to look after you throughout your treatment and any subsequent pregnancy.

Intrauterine Insemination (IUI)

Under this procedure, you will be given tablets or possibly injections to stimulate the ovaries, and you will be monitored very closely by ultrasound. Once you have one or two mature follicles containing eggs and the lining of your womb is thick enough, you will be given another injection to release the eggs. Soon after, your partner's prepared sperm is injected into your womb via a very fine tube.

IUI is often recommended for couples who are experiencing impotence or ejaculation problems or where the male partner's sperm count is low, there's poor motility or the sperm are having difficulties surviving the journey through the cervical mucus. The procedure is usually painless and offers good results (around 15 per cent per cycle of treatment), especially to couples experiencing unexplained infertility or if ovulation problems are an issue.

In vitro fertilization (IVF)

Since the first test-tube baby Louise Brown was born in July 1978, IVF has allowed infertile UK couples to have nearly 70,000 children. In the UK, 30,000 women undergo treatment every year, making IVF one of the most popular fertility treatments available.

The good news is that advances in medical technology are making the entire process more reliable and efficient. The latest screening techniques for eggs and sperm, and the discovery of new drugs to aid egg acceptance has increased the success rate from 15 per cent in the late 1990s to 23 per cent now. Although an overall success rate for conception of around a quarter may sound quite low, this is about the same as in nature.

IVF may be recommended if you are older, you have blocked tubes or you have been unsuccessful with other drug and ART techniques such as ovulation induction or IUI.

IVF treatment given to single women more than doubled in five years, from 215 in 2001 to 536 treatments in 2005.

Q. We have been referred to an IVF clinic miles from our home. Can't we have treatment at a clinic that's not so far away?

A. There is a system called satellite IVF whereby the early stages of treatment are conducted at your local clinic and only the actual placing of the embryos in your body is done at the IVF clinic. This can prove less stressful, time- and cost-consuming. Ask your local unit or check out the HFEA website for a list of licensed clinics offering satellite IVF (**www.hfea.gov.uk**).

Q. After I had my two children, I opted for sterilization as a contraceptive method because my husband would not have a vasectomy. My husband and I divorced several years ago and I am now in a wonderful relationship with a new man who does not have any children from his previous marriage. I would dearly love to have a child with my new partner. It would be the best gift we could ever have. Am I just dreaming?

A. No, you're not dreaming. You can have a reversal after female sterilization. Known in medical terms as a 'reanastomosis after sterilization', the procedure rejoins the severed ends of the fallopian tubes, giving a good chance of achieving a natural pregnancy, with success rates ranging from 50–90 per cent. You don't say which type of sterilization you underwent, but sterilization with clips has the highest chance of being successfully reversed.

MYTH: You can't have IVF treatment if you're over 35 because it won't work.

FACT: The UK NHS-funded treatment is available to women between the ages of 23 and 39 and, in theory, anyone with the means can have private treatment. However, individual clinics in the UK have rules about age limits, which tend to be higher than those of the NHS (up to about 45 years old in general).

The reason an age limit is applied is because female fertility diminishes with age, so if you are using your own eggs, the younger you are, the higher your chances of success. Statistically, one in four women under 30 have babies after IVF, but only one in ten by the age of 40. Nonetheless, IVF can result in a healthy pregnancy for some older women and there are other options to consider such as egg donation (see Chapter 7, page 210).

What should I expect of IVF?

IVF treatment involves several complex steps that may differ slightly from clinic to clinic but which typically involve the following:

- **Boosting egg supply:** Drugs are given to make your ovaries produce more than one egg.

- **Monitoring:** Vaginal ultrasound scans are carried out to monitor your developing eggs. Blood tests are also taken to chart oestrogen levels. At the right time, an injection is given to help your eggs to mature.

- **Egg collection:** Using ultrasound and occasionally laparoscopy (where a small telescope is inserted through a small cut in your abdominal wall), eggs are collected.

- **Sperm collection:** Around the time your eggs are collected, your partner will produce a fresh sperm sample, from which the healthiest and most active sperm will be selected.

- **Fertilization:** Your eggs are mixed with your partner's sperm and left in a laboratory dish. Any that are not fertilized or have fertilized abnormally are discarded.

- **Preparing for pregnancy:** Two days after your eggs have been collected, you are given progesterone via pessaries, injection or gel to help prepare the lining of your womb.

- **Transferring the embryos:** Between two and five days after fertilization, one or two healthy embryos are replaced in your womb.

Remaining embryos may be frozen for future IVF attempts, if they are suitable.

Counting the cost

We are sure that your infertility advisers will discuss with you every aspect of assisted reproductive techniques, including potential costs. Yet, we also understand how, when all you want is a baby, no price can seem too high. However, if you and your partner decide to go ahead with ART, we urge you to give careful consideration to the financial implications before you commit to treatment.

Before you investigate private clinics, did you know that UK citizens may be eligible for treatment on the NHS? From 1 April 2005, the UK government said that all women with appropriate clinical need should have at least one cycle of IVF treatment paid for by the NHS. The only problem is that local health bodies apply their own eligibility criteria, so in reality the vast majority of IVF treatment is still paid for privately.

Nonetheless, NHS treatment is a route worth investigating – the treatment is of the same high standard as going privately, but if time is not on your side, the waiting lists tend to be longer.

To find out if you are eligible for NHS funding, you should consult your doctor for a referral, or contact your Primary Care Trust (England), Local Health Board (Wales), Health Board (Scotland) or Health and Social Services Board (Northern Ireland) direct, and ask for details of their funding policy and who is eligible.

If you are not lucky enough to qualify for NHS treatment, you need to budget for private treatment and this is costly. Prices vary considerably depending on where you live and the clinic you choose, but a typical cost of a cycle of IVF treatment alone is approximately £3,000 and you also have to pay for the costs of consultation, drugs and tests on top of that.

Q. What is natural cycle IVF?

A. There are no fertility drugs used in natural IVF. Rather the one egg that you release during your normal monthly cycle is collected and fertilized. This avoids any drug side effects, the risk of a multiple pregnancy and, because your ovaries have not been artificially stimulated, they don't need to rest after IVF, so allowing you to try again sooner if your treatment is unsuccessful.

Freezing and storing embryos

During IVF treatment, you sometimes end up with more healthy embryos than can be used during that cycle of treatment (under the UK Human Fertilisation and Embryology Authority – HFEA – rules, only two embryos can be transferred if you're under 40 and three embryos if you're 40 or over). Most clinics will then offer you the opportunity of having these 'excess' healthy embryos frozen and stored for future use. Embryos can be stored for up to five years or sometimes ten years, and in exceptional circumstances, this period can be extended still further.

One of the advantages of this option is that if you decide to have another cycle of IVF, you avoid the lengthy and sometimes difficult stages of drug treatment, egg stimulation and collection. However, your chances of conceiving using frozen embryos is slightly lower than with a fresh embryo. The good news is that frozen embryos are not affected by how long they have been stored, so this will not affect your chances of becoming pregnant.

Donating your embryos

Whether you now have the family you want or you have decided to discontinue IVF treatment, if you still have embryos in frozen storage, you will be offered the opportunity to donate them, either to another person (see Chapter 7, page 214) or for use in research into advancing IVF technology or stem cell studies.

This is a decision that only you and your partner can make, although counselling and advice about the implications will be available. Rest assured that your embryos cannot be used in this way without your written consent.

Q. What is the problem with having a multiple pregnancy?

A. If you are carrying more than one baby, the pregnancy and birth are more prone to complications for both you and your babies. The higher the number of babies, the higher the associated risks.

Gamete Intra-Fallopian Transfer (GIFT)

GIFT was one of the first ARTs and it is still popular today. Your eggs and sperm are collected in exactly the same way as for IVF. The healthiest are then selected, mixed together outside the body and immediately transferred back into your fallopian tube so that fertilization can happen as it would normally. GIFT can only be used if your fallopian tubes are not blocked or damaged, but it can help in many cases of unexplained infertility or if the man has a low sperm count or low motility.

Male fertility issues

The progress made in the field of ART since the late 1990s is truly remarkable, to the extent that it is now possible, using micromanipulation, for a couple to have a healthy baby even though the man has a very low sperm count and virtually no motile sperm.

Under this advanced procedure known as 'intra-cytoplasmic sperm injection' (ICSI), one of your prepared ova (eggs) is placed under a microscope and injected directly with an individual sperm that has been collected from your partner's semen specimen or even surgically taken directly from his testicles (termed TESE, testicular sperm extraction) or from his epididymis, the tubes that collect the semen from the testes (percutaneous epididymal sperm aspiration – PESA or micro-epididymal sperm aspiration – MESA).

This advanced micromanipulation procedure has given hope to couples who, only a few years ago, would have had no chance of conceiving a child because the man had such a low sperm count or motility.

Finding a private clinic

Your doctor and the local hospital infertility consultant will be able to give you some advice if you decide to look at private treatment for assisted conception.

However, if you are doing your own research, or want to spread your net wider, the government regulatory body that inspects all UK clinics and licenses and monitors all human embryo research conducted in the UK, the Human Fertilisation and Embryology Authority (HFEA), offers an interactive clinic search facility on its website (**www.hfea.gov.uk**) and the site also gives advice on how to make your choice.

There are currently 85 HFEA-licensed infertility clinics in the UK, 52 of which also treat NHS patients. The HFEA recommends that, among other things, you consider the following when making your decision:

- **Location:** Treatment may be required at anti-social hours so distance from your home and ease of access should be considered.

- **Cost:** If you are paying privately, comparing prices between clinics is important.

- **Specializations:** Some clinics may have special interests and expertise in specific treatments.

- **Personal recommendation:** Can the clinic put you in touch with other patients?

- **Privacy:** What provisions are there for the protection of your privacy and dignity at the clinic?

- **Support networks:** What sort of support groups or counselling does the clinic offer and is it free or an additional cost?

- **Rules and regulations:** Does the clinic have any selection criteria for patients or restrictions such as age or sexual orientation?

- **Success rate:** Be wary of making a decision solely on 'live birth rates' as they are called, because these are incredibly difficult to interpret. For example, clinics that only treat younger couples will usually have better success rates than a clinic that takes older couples or couples who need complicated treatment.

- **Embryo transfer:** Clinics can replace two embryos at each IVF attempt, or three if you are aged 40 or over (and using your own eggs). Some clinics prefer to replace one embryo to reduce the risks associated with multiple pregnancy, and to freeze any remaining embryos for use in the future.

Seeking help abroad

There are no official statistics for the numbers of women travelling abroad from the UK for fertility treatment, but the website **www.fertilityfriends.co.uk**, which shares information about foreign clinics, receives more than 2 million hits a month. You might even have looked into this option yourself. Some of the reasons given by prospective parents for undergoing treatment abroad include:

- Long UK waiting lists.

- Less than 25 per cent of all IVF treatment in the UK is funded by the NHS and the costs for private treatment is high.

- The cost of IVF treatment in countries such as Hungary and Slovenia is around 2,400 euros (£1,608) – about half the cost in the UK.

- Stocks of eggs and sperm in clinics across the UK have declined since legislation ending anonymous egg and sperm donation came into force in 2005.

- Countries such as Spain, India, Russia, the US and a number of eastern European countries, still guarantee donor anonymity so stocks are plentiful, which is obviously attractive to women requiring egg donation.

- In some countries, up to five embryos can be implanted (in the UK no more than three embryos can be implanted at a time – and moves are afoot to limit this to one), increasing the chance of success but also the chance of a multiple pregnancy.

- Few UK fertility clinics will treat women over 45, yet in Italy, over-60s are treated.

However, you should know that the HFEA is concerned that if you go abroad, you may be treated in unregulated clinics that are not as rigorous in practices, such as screening donors for example, as they are in the UK. It also cautions that you may not have access to counselling after treatment, and that you may be offered dangerous treatments, such as implanting five embryos, with all the inherent risks of multiple pregnancy.

How will you know what's best for you?

Once again, we have given you a vast amount of information and we know that it is a lot to take on board. Hopefully, you will re-read parts of this chapter in bite-sized chunks, so that you are confident that you know what each of the options entails.

Although we have given you the facts to digest at your own pace, we also recommend that you discuss your next move not only with your partner, but also with your doctor, the medical team at your infertility unit and perhaps even seek the views and experiences of other couples who have been through the process of choosing treatment options (Chapter 5 gives details of support networks).

Some couples decide that they do not want to put themselves through further tests or treatment and, although they would still love to have a baby, they prefer to wait and see what happens over time and without intervention. Others are keen to start treatment without delay. Whatever you and your partner decide, it has to feel right for you both. **Don't let anyone pressurize you** into a course of action that you don't want. Don't worry, you will tend to know instinctively what is right for you both.

If you decide to pursue a course of treatment, whether it is conventional or complementary or an integrated mixture of both, then may we suggest that you decide with your partner what your short-term goal is? Perhaps it's to correct a physical problem such as a blocked tube and then to continue trying to conceive naturally, or it may be to complete one cycle of the most appropriate ART.

At this point, you may also find it beneficial to reconfirm your long-term goal of having a baby – but to be more specific. For example, are you prepared to explore every treatment option or are you happy to try drug treatment but prefer not to undergo ART? These are highly individual decisions but goal-setting like this can help you both to feel that you are doing all that you can right now and that you are heading in the right direction.

I have had unexplained infertility for approximately four years. We have been having conventional treatment for three years and, after two failed IVF cycles and one tragic miscarriage, I turned to a natural preconceptual care charity, and we followed their advice. We had hair analysis and embarked on the full supplement programme. I had already changed our diet to eliminate all refined sugar, cake, aspartame, chocolate and caffeine, and now we filtered our water and tried our best to buy organic. Anyway, we now have two wonderful baby boys, conceived naturally.

Sarah

We have a son Joshua, nine years in the coming, three types of fertility treatment, eleventh time lucky, but first time IVF successful and YES it was all worth it!

I suppose what I'm trying to say is, please don't give up. Our son is our miracle. Joshua is now nine months old, weighs 16lb, and doing fantastic. Without the belief that one day it will happen, we would have given up. My husband's continuous support and encouragement gave me that belief. So go that extra mile.

Melanie

5

Emotional lifelines

You have come an amazing distance since the start of this book, even though it may not feel like it at times. First, you've faced the fact that you may have difficulties in conceiving and second, you've taken the positive step of deciding to do something about it, even if it is simply reading this book and becoming informed.

In many ways, you may feel relieved that you are now seeking advice or are thinking about undergoing tests to discover the cause, if any, for the delay in becoming pregnant. Or you may be further down the fertility road and you are already seeking treatment of the kind we discussed in Chapter 4.

Irrespective of where you find yourself along this path, going through tests and/or fertility treatment is bound to trigger all kinds of emotions for you. There is the relief, hope and excitement that follow the decision to take action, the nervous anticipation of receiving results, the joy of success or the disappointment of a setback.

As we discussed in Chapter 2, it is perfectly natural to experience a full range of emotions at this time. While each person's situation is unique and everyone copes in his or her own way with the emotional and psychological pressure of tests and treatment, we want to remind you again that you are not alone in feeling the way you do, and there are always loved ones, friends, support networks or professionals who can and will be supportive.

Working things out as a couple

Fertility treatment can be an extremely stressful experience for both you and your partner and it can put a strain on even the best relationship. If you have been used to talking over your worries, concerns and feelings with each other, well done because you're already in a strong position to cope with the welter of emotions thrown up by fertility treatment.

Remember to try to make time for each other and for the things that you enjoy, especially those things that are completely unrelated to fertility issues and babies, and consciously ask for or offer the support that each of you needs. Sharing your feelings really can help.

Bear in mind that, however good your relationship and your communication, it is easy, under the pressure of tests and treatment, to lose sight sometimes of the fact that you are on the same side. We are all quick to lash out at the ones we love the most when we are feeling tense and angry, but don't forget that you are both striving for the same result and that you will get through this together. If you can, also make an effort to forgive and forget any outbursts since you both know these are simply a reaction to the pressure of what you're currently experiencing and that it will pass.

By the same token, try to resist the temptation to blame the other person for what is happening to you. **No one is guilty and it is no one's fault.** It can only be divisive to lay the blame at your partner's door, or vice versa.

Some women feel that they shoulder a disproportionate amount of the physical discomfort of infertility treatment since they have to undergo almost all of the invasive investigations and medical interventions. Whereas we can completely identify with your reaction, we also know that many men express feelings of guilt that their partner has to go through the treatment, especially if something is wrong with their sperm, for example. You and your partner might like to discuss this inevitable imbalance rather than leaving it unsaid and as a slightly uncomfortable tacit agreement between you. Getting any resentment into the open, however small, in a calm way is definitely healthier than harbouring grievances in private or letting them slip out in an argument.

Talking things through and trying to see your fertility situation from the other partner's perspective is not only very beneficial now but it can also bring a new intensity to your relationship that is based on mutual respect and understanding.

Support for couples

If the stress of your situation has created or exacerbated problems within your relationship that you do not feel able to heal on your own, you might want to seek some additional help to sort the problems out. Relate is a UK counselling charity that works with couples experiencing relationship difficulties. Although they do not specialize in infertility, they can give relationship guidance either to you and your partner individually, or as a couple (see Part 5, Chapter 12 for details).

Instant tension release

Aromatic essential oils from plants have been used for thousands of years for their healing and medicinal value, but also for their capacity to relax you. Treat yourself to a relaxing aromatherapy massage when things are getting on top of you, and keep some oils at home for inhalation or to use in a relaxing bath as part of your self-care strategy.

For an instant pick-me-up when you're feeling stressed, put a couple of drops of essential oil on a tissue or handkerchief and inhale whenever you get the chance. Some of the best aromas for combating stress are:

- cedarwood
- lavender
- roman chamomile
- petitgrain
- sandalwood
- sweet marjoram.

Note: Some essential oils are not recommended for use during pregnancy, so if you suspect you may be pregnant, avoid using these stress-busting oils, or consult a herbalist or aromatherapist first.

Dealing with your feelings

Since you have been looking for answers as to why you're not pregnant yet, you have probably felt a renewed sense of hope and direction and we are glad for you. Being in the hands of a good doctor or clinic can be hugely reassuring, too. Yet undergoing investigations and waiting for results can also be emotionally demanding.

If you're already into the treatment phase, you'll find more information about coping with your emotions later in this chapter (see page 148), but for those not at that stage, here are some of the more common and very normal reactions felt by many couples as they go through evaluation and diagnosis:

- Feeling out of control – 'It's as if doctors, tests and schedules rule your life.'

- Isolation – not wanting to explain the infertility testing to friends and family.

- Lack of privacy due to the invasive nature of the tests.

- Lack of sexuality – what was fun and spontaneous is now scheduled and monitored by doctors.

- Shock and numbness.

- Feeling misunderstood by others who have children.

- Anger and disappointment and feelings of 'Why us?'

How to cope with your feelings

We know this is a trying time but you will come through the other side sooner than you think. In the meantime, here are a few strategies to get you through this phase:

- Find out as much as you can about infertility, its causes and treatment, both by reading this and other books, visiting our recommended websites and speaking to your fertility experts.

- Keep communicating with your partner about your feelings and anxieties.

- Be there for each other at low times.

- Know that you will have times when you feel low or anxious (see above), and don't beat yourself up for feeling that way. It's not weak or self-pitying, it's a natural reaction and you must do what's best for you to get through these occasions.

- Allow yourself some time of peace and solitude so you can get your thoughts and feelings straight in your own mind.

- Try talking to trusted friends and relatives and, if you can, accept their offers of support.

- Find a support group or someone who has been through this (see Infertility Network UK in Part 5, page 304).

MYTH: Some stress is good for you.

FACT: Meeting a challenge or doing something exciting is good for you. It stretches your boundaries and puts you under manageable pressure, but stress is different. Stress is when we feel overstretched and unable to cope. Everyone has their own stress threshold, of course, but when you are trying to sort out your fertility issues, you do not need additional stress or pressure in your life if you can help it.

How other couples with fertility issues can help

If you choose not to involve family and friends or if you worry that those you confide in are beginning to grow tired of hearing your concerns, you will find that other couples experiencing infertility can be a constant and reliable source of support. They will always be there for you as a listening and supportive ear. They will continue to understand when others just can't, or haven't the time or energy.

It helps if you can have regular contact with other couples who you know are taking a long time to conceive or who are going through investigations or treatment, or with a support group in your area. In fact, most clinics have patient support groups set up by and for patients themselves. If not, your doctor or fertility team will almost certainly know of local groups. There is also plenty of support on the internet or telephone too, which can be a good alternative for those couples daunted by groups (see Part 5).

Unless you've experienced infertility, you can't really understand what it's like. It can be such a relief and an enormous support to share your feelings with someone who really knows what you're talking about.

Finding local support

Infertility Network UK (see page 304) has a number of volunteers who act as local contacts and who often have a wealth of knowledge about local infertility services, and can suggest someone you can talk to in your area. Many also run local support groups where you can meet others face to face – people who are in a similar situation to yourself.

The organization has regional organizers throughout the UK who support these groups and help volunteers to set up new groups in areas of need. These groups not only provide people experiencing infertility with a chance to meet others in their area who are in the same situation but there are also local guest speakers for a variety of infertility-related subjects. Such groups are an invaluable source of support. They provide a vehicle for sharing information on local services. For more information on groups in your area or if you would like more details on Infertility Network UK's services, go to **www.infertilitynetwork.com**.

Taking time out from fertility

On occasion, it can feel as if trying for a baby is the sole focus of your life, and that's not good for you, your partner or your relationships. So why not take time out occasionally and make some time for activities or things that are completely unrelated to fertility or conceiving. Try:

- catching up with old friends

- putting aside a night to go out with your partner and make a rule that you will not discuss tests or treatment

- putting yourself forward for a new project at work – something to throw yourself into

- having sex for the fun of it, whenever you like, wherever you like – and definitely at the wrong time of the month!

- going on a weekend break and trying a new activity that you've never tried before: quad biking, water-colour painting – whatever appeals.

How you might feel during treatment

By the time you undergo treatment, you may feel that your fertility issues are dominating your lives. You are also likely to feel pretty tired a lot of the time, especially if you are going through in vitro fertilization (IVF) treatment, and this can make you more susceptible to your emotions.

At the same time as feeling frustrated with the demands of infertility treatment, you may also be feeling excited and hopeful. Try to hold on to these positive thoughts and don't worry too much about conflicting emotions: they are natural and very common at this time too. Other common emotions and reactions that couples in treatment have shared with us include:

- **Frustration** – at having to invest so much time, energy, emotion and money in treatment.

- **A strong sense of injustice** – it shouldn't be happening to us.

- **Indignity and vulnerability** – particularly acute in women, because of the intrusive and intimate nature of treatment.

- **Lack of control and emotional turmoil** – common to both partners as doctors appear to be taking over, but the hormonal effects of infertility drugs can amplify these feelings in women.

- **Sensitivity** – people seem inadvertently to say the wrong or hurtful things.

- **Self-doubt** – 'have we done all we can to have a baby?'

- **Financial worry** – can we afford the cost of treatment?

- **Reduced sexuality** – lovemaking is no longer an expression of mutual intimacy.

You have been through so much already to get to the point of treatment, that it is easy to forget to acknowledge what you have achieved so far. Although treatment can feel like the ultimate point on a long journey, it is really just the beginning, whatever the future holds for you.

Success may not be achieved on the first attempt. It may require time, considerable effort and repeated attempts, but try to remember that there is always hope. A successful resolution may be just around the corner for you.

Trying to hold on to these positive thoughts can make the strain of the treatment phase more bearable. Here are some more strategies that other couples have found helpful in coping with the demands of infertility treatment:

- Try not to dwell on the immediate treatment but focus on your long-term goals.

- Don't bottle up your feelings – let it out if you've reached your limit.

- Remember to follow the self-help techniques from Chapter 4 (page 98). If you are in the best of health, you will be better able to cope with the treatment and the ensuing emotions.

- Complementary therapies and relaxation techniques can help ease the stress.

- Don't wait for 'failure'. You have various treatment options open to you at all times, so you don't have to exhaust one route before turning to the next. For example, while waiting for IVF results, do some research on egg donation (see Chapter 7, page 210), or even put your name on the list. You can always take your name off the list if you get pregnant. This helps to keep you focused and motivated.

- Count your successes and feel proud of yourself. If you've managed to lose the 12 lb (5 kg) needed to begin your first IVF cycle, that's great. Congratulate yourself on taking another important step.

- Seek emotional support and guidance from a counsellor or support group.

Q. Once we've started with tests and investigations, will we be able to get out of the system if we decide against treatment?

A. You can stop at any stage of the investigations, or even treatment, and your decision will be fine with your doctor and fertility team. Whether to have treatment or to carry on trying naturally for a baby is a highly personal decision and you must do what is right for you and your partner. Some couples choose to have tests to verify whether or not there is an obstacle to conception. If there is no identifiable reason for the delay in getting pregnant, then they opt to let things happen in their own time. Others learn of a possible cause for their infertility but decide that treatment is not an option for them. The decision is always and firmly yours as a couple, and yours alone. Nobody will pressurize you into undertaking treatment that you are not happy with.

Counselling

Although you and your partner can undoubtedly support each other by talking through your feelings, and trusted friends and family can also help, sometimes it helps to talk to an expert trained in fertility issues who is experienced in helping couples to process their emotions.

Many clinics offer counselling services to couples before, during and after fertility treatment and, if a counsellor is not available on site, they should be able to give you information on independent services in your area.

Support counselling aims to give emotional support at times of particular stress during treatment, for example, when you are awaiting results or if a treatment has not been successful.

MYTH: You only seek counselling if you're weak and can't solve your own problems.

FACT: Infertility is not a mental problem. You are not neurotic or psychotic and you are certainly not weak if you seek help and advice. Infertility can cause you to experience a confusion of emotions and you may benefit from talking these feelings through with someone trained to understand all aspects of what you are undergoing.

It's chiefly used to help you to work through your emotions. However, as we have already discussed, infertility can be a turbulent process that highlights all sorts of different issues. Perhaps it makes you think about a painful experience from your past or you may be starting to feel unduly worried about treatment. In these situations, **therapeutic counselling** might be better because it shows you how to work through difficult issues and to deal with the impact that infertility can have on your life and your relationships.

What to expect

Your clinic should provide you with contact details for a counsellor. Some clinics offer a free service, but not all. We recommend that you ask right at the beginning of your relationship about what their counselling service comprises, if it is an additional cost and how much it might be.

You may prefer to find your own counsellor outside of the clinic, or you can contact voluntary infertility organizations that offer counselling support and networks. Counselling is not right for everyone, but in the majority of cases it proves to be beneficial. Here are some of the things that counselling might give you:

- A chance to talk candidly in confidence and without being judged.

- An opportunity to explore your feelings and any sensitive issues that are troubling you.

- Support in reaching your own decisions, finding your own solutions and ways of coping.

- Help in understanding factors that may be contributing to your difficulties.

Q. What if I don't want to see the clinic's counsellor? Can we still have treatment?

A. You may have your own reasons for not wanting to use the clinic's counselling service. Perhaps you are already seeing a therapist, or maybe you feel the support of your partner, friends and relatives is all the help you need. Whatever your reason, that's fine. Taking advantage of the clinic's counselling service is not compulsory although it is recommended. You could consider attending one session to judge for yourself whether or not you might find some benefit in attending another session.

Going forward

We have now come to the end of Part 2, and we hope the information has been useful to you. We know there's a lot to take in but there's no rush: take your time and re-read it as often as you like.

When you're ready, you can move on to Part 3, where we look at what you might expect in the longer term, which may involve developing strategies to deal with prolonged treatment. We also explore what might lie beyond treatment, whether that involves the uncertainties of being pregnant, looking at alternative ways to have a family life, or making a conscious decision to stop treatment when the time is right.

It hurt so much that my mum and friends kept belittling what we were going through because we already had a child. I know I'm lucky to have such a beautiful daughter but I wanted another child so badly. Just because we'd chosen to go through ICSI for a second child, it didn't make it any less difficult. I just wanted them to listen and be there for me, not to judge me or tell me I should be grateful because I have my daughter.

Suzy

Initially, I felt that my body had let me down. Over the next eight years, I swung between feeling utterly defeated to being determined, from resentful to hopeful. I hated feeling left out because we didn't have a baby. Our parents didn't know how to help but Pete's mum called a helpline for relatives of people with infertility and that was really useful. Our first attempt at ICSI failed but on the third attempt, using ICSI and assisted hatching, I conceived our son, Joshua.

Trisha

The expert's view

Some of our work involves helping people to talk about their experiences and to understand the underlying issues, which makes it easier for them to find ways to cope or sort out problems.

It's not surprising that infertility affects the rest of people's lives. It's pretty hard to face friends with children, or to deal with talk at work about families or with someone going on maternity leave. Within a relationship, too, infertility can cause a huge amount of stress.

We offer people a safe space where they can focus on their problems and be supported in finding their own solutions. Often, just sharing feelings with someone outside their circle of friends and relations brings a sense of relief.

Many of our patients see counselling as a useful way of preparing for treatment – as an extra source of support and stress management during it. It can be especially important for those faced with a negative pregnancy test or if there are problems with the pregnancy itself.

A skilled counsellor can play a vital role in enabling couples to deal with the emotional challenges of these difficult experiences.

**Jennifer Hunt,
Senior Infertility Counsellor,
Hammersmith Hospital**

Part 3:
Long-term
Challenges and
Future Hopes

6

Successful conception
and a healthy pregnancy

So far, we've discussed the practical steps you can take with regards to your fertility situation. These range from the investigations that might identify possible reasons why you haven't got pregnant to the various treatment options that are on offer. We have also looked at how you might be feeling during this investigation and treatment stage of your journey. Now we need to take a more long-term view of your situation and the possible outcomes of any actions you might have taken. However, take a moment to acknowledge that you have already achieved a great deal, even though, as yet, you have not reached your ultimate goal of having a baby. You've taken constructive action to discover what, if anything, might be causing your problems and you've armed yourself with detailed information about causes and treatments for infertility. You are in a position where you can make an informed decision about how to deal with your own unique situation.

Whether you have decided upon the 'wait and see' option or have actively pursued one or several of the treatment choices, you can rightly feel that you're doing everything within your power to make conception happen.

We are at the stage of the book where we are going to focus on several topics that may affect you as you move through and beyond the investigation and treatment phase. First, in this chapter, we look at what happens if treatment is successful. We explore ways of getting used to the idea of being pregnant, the practical steps involved in your continued care, and the mixed emotions your successful conception may bring. Pregnancy is a new and different journey from the one we have travelled together so far, but in this chapter we discuss the inevitable ups and downs that you may experience along the way, and offer help and support if you need it.

In Chapter 7, we'll investigate ways to stick at it when treatments are unsuccessful and give advice on how to stay positive and focused. In addition, there are plenty of suggested strategies to help you through the stressful periods of continued treatment and tips to help you deal with the tensions of awaiting results.

Finally, in Chapter 8, we look at whether or not the alternatives to giving birth, such as adoption or surrogacy, might be right for you. We also explore the thorny issue of knowing when to say enough is enough, and there will be advice to help you if and when you decide the time is right for such a decision. If you so choose, we'll help you to plan for a full and rewarding life as a couple beyond treatment.

How do you know if you're pregnant?

If you are having fertility treatment, most clinics offer a pregnancy test a couple of weeks after your treatment, although some couples prefer to self-test at home anyway. If you use a home-testing kit, read the instructions very carefully because different brands vary in how they show a positive result. Whether you get the news from your clinic or whether you self-test, if you get a positive test result, that's great news and we're delighted for you both.

We understand that making the transition from being a fertility patient to an expectant mother may not be quite as straightforward and joyous as you'd imagined but don't worry, it's perfectly normal to have a mixed reaction to the good news. We have some suggestions to help you to make the transition as smoothly as possible so that both you and your partner can relax and enjoy the pregnancy and the prospect of your new baby.

> *MYTH: A pregnancy test kit never shows positive if you are not pregnant.*
>
> **FACT:** Home pregnancy test kits are now very accurate and can give a correct reading at a couple of weeks. However, if you are over-eager (which is understandable) and test too early, you could get a false result. Whatever the test result, whether it's negative or a weak positive, if you tested before the recommended time, it's worth doing another test at a later date to double-check.

What do you do next?

After any kind of assisted reproduction technology (ART) treatment, if you get a positive pregnancy test result from a home-testing kit, you should let the clinic know so they can enter the data on the UK Human Fertilisation and Embryology Authority (HFEA) register. Your fertility team will also want to discuss with you whether or not you need any further treatment such as progesterone suppositories, aspirin or even heparin. The clinic may then offer you an ultrasound scan in the early weeks of your pregnancy to make sure your baby is developing normally and to see if you're carrying twins.

However, do double-check, because not all clinics offer this service.

After the initial scans from your clinic (or straightaway if continued care is not an option), you'll need to visit your doctor to discuss and arrange your antenatal care and birth options. He or she will then book a visit to the hospital where you'll meet the midwives and doctors who are going to look after you and your baby during the pregnancy. If you're going to use private health care, you'll need to make an appointment with a private consultant – either your doctor or your fertility clinic may be able to suggest someone in your area.

Some large hospitals in the UK, whether they are National Health Service (NHS) or private, have both infertility and maternity units on site, and if you're going to be transferred from one unit to the next, your notes should automatically be passed over at the same time so that your history is known. If this is not the case, then it's up to you to tell the doctors and midwives of your antenatal team about your fertility treatment.

Antenatal care doesn't really kick in until around the twelfth week of pregnancy and, as women with fertility issues find out about their pregnancy very early on, this is a long time to be without support. Some fertility clinics encourage you to stay in touch in the first few weeks and their counsellors will probably still be available to you if you want someone to talk to at this stage.

Don't be surprised if you're feeling slightly numb, confused or just not as overjoyed as you expected to be. This is perfectly normal. It takes time to adjust and there are people who can help you through this transitional period, as we'll see in the next section of this chapter. It's also worth knowing that many expectant women, irrespective of whether or not they've had fertility difficulties, go through a mixture of emotions on discovering that they are pregnant. It's really not unusual and nothing to worry about.

MYTH: If you have problems getting pregnant, then you'll have problems being pregnant.

FACT: This is just **not** the case. The risk of miscarriage or ectopic pregnancy is slightly higher than with a normal pregnancy after fertility treatment, but in the majority of cases, the way you conceive bears no relation to the type of pregnancy you might have. You may suffer morning sickness, etc. or you may sail through without a symptom. Let's hope it's the latter.

Culture clash

If you've been through fertility treatment, you will be used to being closely monitored and carefully scrutinized so it can come as a surprise to find yourself in the more laid-back hands of the antenatal care services where appointments might be months apart and you may see a different face each time.

Try not to worry unduly. You are in good hands; it's simply a different approach. If this change in care style leaves you feeling unnerved or too isolated, think about joining an antenatal group such as the UK's National Childbirth Trust (NCT) or a support group like Assisted Conception Babies (AceBabes) (see Part 5 for details) so that you can talk about your anxieties and fears and share your experiences with other mothers-to-be.

Staying healthy for you and your baby

To have a good, full-term pregnancy and to improve the prospects of a healthy baby, it is important that you take care of yourself by:

- eating a nutritionally rich diet

- getting plenty of rest and regular exercise

- taking folic acid supplements

- avoiding known miscarriage triggers such as alcohol and nicotine

- being as relaxed as possible and trying not to worry too much.

Should you be feeling more delighted?

The initial exhilaration of a positive pregnancy test is often followed by a mass of conflicting emotions. You may feel strangely removed from reality, and the baby might seem almost separate from you. Conversely, you may be preoccupied with your body and conscious of every little twinge or strange sensation. It is natural to feel cautious about celebrating so early in your pregnancy, while perhaps another part of you wants to shout your news from the rooftops. All these reactions are understandable and you should try to accept your feelings, whatever they are, without becoming too concerned.

We realize that if you have become used to handling the difficulties of delayed conception and fertility treatment, it can be hard to adjust to the news that you are pregnant, and it can also be difficult to know who to turn to for support if you need it.

Some women who become pregnant tell us that they don't feel at home in the world of antenatal clinics and yet they no longer belong in their infertility circle. They are conscious that they don't want to upset the friends they've made through their fertility treatment and who are perhaps still experiencing difficulties in conceiving. It's as if you fall between two stools, and this sudden lack of support can be alarming. Yet there are people who can fill the gap. Your clinic may be able to put you in touch with other women who have had a baby or are expecting a baby after fertility treatment who will be able to empathize with how you are feeling.

AceBabes is a charity in the UK that has a special section for couples who are expecting a baby after fertility treatment. It's called Bump Buddies, and the aim is to help couples get in touch with others who are at the same stage of pregnancy so that they can be there for one another (see Part 5, Chapter 12 for details).

Alternatively, one of the talking therapies that we discussed in Chapter 4 could be an invaluable bridge and support until such time as your antenatal care starts in earnest. Or you might prefer to talk to family and friends, although it's not always easy to gauge when it's best to tell them your good news.

> **MYTH:** *Sexual intercourse could jeopardize the pregnancy.*
>
> **FACT:** Unless you are expressly told otherwise by your fertility consultant, there is no reason why you can't enjoy sexual relations during your pregnancy. It will not harm the baby and it can be wonderful to rediscover sexual intimacy as a couple after the intrusion of fertility treatment. However, some couples report a loss of libido during a pregnancy, irrespective of how the baby was conceived, and a few women are so exhausted both emotionally and physically after undergoing fertility treatment that their sexual interest is virtually non-existent. Ultimately, it's your body from start to finish and you know better than anyone whether or not sex feels right for you or not, but as far as medical advice is concerned, feel free to indulge.

When to tell loved ones your good news

You may be so elated that you want to share your joy with your loved ones without delay, but you may also feel that you'd rather wait until you've had your first scan, or even got past the 12-week point before you tell anyone.

There is no right or wrong way to handle this. Whatever feels best for you and your partner is the only guidance we can give. What we can say is that your friends and family will be delighted for you both but they may not realize that you are experiencing some mixed emotions.

Perhaps they may express surprise that you cannot simply 'relax and enjoy the pregnancy'. Once again, how much you confide in your friends and family is down to the individual relationships but it may be worth pointing out that you wish to guard against possible disappointment at this early stage of the pregnancy by not being too overtly excited – and that should silence any of the 'This is what you wanted, isn't it?' conversations.

Once you are pregnant, having been through so much to get here, you may feel that you have no right to express any complaints about the discomforts associated with pregnancy. Let us reassure you right now that even though this pregnancy is very precious to you, that does not lessen the discomforts of morning sickness or aching legs, for example, and you are just as likely as the next pregnant woman to have the occasional negative thought or experience in your pregnancy. Don't feel you cannot voice these feelings just because you've been through infertility treatment. We suggest you share how you feel with other pregnant women, friends and family, whether it is good, bad or indifferent, because that's natural.

Q. I'm 38 years old and pregnant after using donor eggs from a 30-year-old woman in my fertility treatment. My antenatal team are recommending an amniocentesis because of my age but is this necessary?

A. The risk of chromosomal abnormalities, such as Down's syndrome, increase with the age of the mother (and ipso facto her eggs), so women over the age of 37 are offered the amniocentesis procedure, which withdraws fluid from the uterus to screen for chromosomal abnormalities. However, since your baby was conceived using the egg of a 30 year old, the baby is not at increased risk and the test is unnecessary in your case.

Instances such as yours highlight why it is important to think carefully about how much you disclose about your fertility treatment to your antenatal team when you transfer from your fertility clinic, as some information affects the advice you are given.

Ectopic pregnancy

This is when the embryo starts to grow outside the uterus, usually in the fallopian tube, but occasionally in the ovary or cervix. With ART, even though the embryo may be placed in your uterus, there is still a risk of an ectopic pregnancy and that risk is slightly higher if you have had damaged tubes or a previous ectopic pregnancy. Tell-tale symptoms to watch out for include:

- vaginal bleeding

- pain in the abdomen (usually on one side only)

- fainting

- pain in the shoulder (on the same side as the abdominal pain).

If you have any of these symptoms, you should get medical advice straightaway. An ultrasound scan and/or blood tests will help confirm the diagnosis. In acute cases, the fallopian tube bursts causing severe pain, shock, a weak but rapid pulse and falling blood pressure. These cases, thankfully rare, require immediate admission to hospital and emergency surgery.

However, almost 60 per cent of women who have had an ectopic pregnancy become pregnant again, while around 30 per cent of women choose to avoid further pregnancy.

When things go wrong

Perhaps the most common worry for women who finally get pregnant after experiencing infertility is the fear of miscarriage. You've spent so long waiting for this pregnancy and now you may feel beset with worries – wishing the first 12 weeks were over so you can reach the safer waters of the second trimester (pregnancy is divided into three phases of roughly three months each, known as the first, second and third trimester).

It may help to know that every pregnant woman fears losing her baby, but we understand that this anxiety is magnified when you know that you may not find it easy to get pregnant again. These worries are natural and very common and, although you may find it hard, you should try to relax and enjoy your pregnancy rather than wishing it away.

More than a million babies around the world have now been born as a result of assisted reproduction treatments such as in vitro fertilization (IVF) and the chances are that you will give birth to a wonderful, healthy baby.

However, we cannot rule out the slight chance of problems, and very sadly there are occasions when a pregnancy ends in miscarriage. If it should unfortunately happen to you, it's important that you and your partner are able to address your feelings of loss, and allow yourselves a period of bereavement before trying to conceive again. It may be painful to discuss, but it can be extremely valuable to talk about your loss to your midwife, health visitor, fertility counsellor or family doctor, or contact the Miscarriage Association in the UK (see Part 5, page 304) which has trained counsellors and support groups.

MYTH: Too much sport or a fall can cause a miscarriage.

FACT: Pregnant women are sometimes afraid that if they should have a fall or over-exert themselves physically they may miscarry, but this is not generally cause for concern. The baby is extremely well cushioned inside the placenta and the womb, and should be perfectly safe. However, if you do a lot of high impact activities such as horse riding, running or aerobics, you might like to consider a lower impact alternative until after the birth if this gives you greater peace of mind.

Your partner may need support too

Since it's the woman who goes through the physical process of miscarriage and undergoes any medical intervention (she may need an operation known as dilation and curettage – D&C – to clean her womb), the focus of attention tends to fall on you. Yet your partner can be just as devastated – both mentally and emotionally – so try to ensure that you both seek support.

It is also common for the man to feel the need to 'be strong' for you, and consequently not show how badly he is hurting, which may appear as being uncaring to you. So try to be honest with each other and share your feelings, as you have done throughout your fertility journey so far.

Small consolation though it may be, try to keep in mind that you are not alone. One-fifth of all women have a miscarriage, so there is probably someone you know, who probably has a family, who has been through this and might be able to help you. And, just because you've had one miscarriage, it doesn't mean it will happen again: recurrent miscarriage (defined as three consecutive miscarriages) affects only about 1 per cent of women.

Q. I am 29 years old and expecting twins after successful IVF treatment. Am I more likely to miscarry because they were conceived artificially?

A. Any pregnancy carries a 15 per cent chance of miscarriage. Following fertility treatment, the risk is slightly higher at around 15–20 per cent. This is largely because the pregnancy tests are carried out earlier in the pregnancy for women who have fertility treatment, when the pregnancy is much more vulnerable. For women who conceive without help, what is dismissed as a 'late period' may in fact be a very early miscarriage where the embryo fails to implant. In addition, the statistics are slightly higher after fertility treatment because the risk of miscarriage rises with the mother's age and, on average, women who undergo fertility treatment tend to be older than women who conceive naturally.

As you are expecting twins, you may need more scans or appointments at the hospital, but rest assured that your antenatal team will be giving you the best care possible and that statistically you are well placed to have a healthy pregnancy.

Possible causes of miscarriage

Age – the risk of miscarriage in women under 40 is 5 per cent. In over forties, it rises to 23 per cent.

Hormonal – if you have hormone irregularities, you are at greater risk of miscarriage.

Genetic abnormality – about half of all early miscarriages occur because of chance chromosome abnormalities so the foetus fails to implant in the uterine wall.

Weight – it is important to fall within the recommended weight band for your height. Being either under- or overweight can lead to an increased risk of miscarriage.

Environmental hazards – both smoking and drinking can adversely affect the quality of a man's sperm. This in turn can lead to a genetic abnormality if such sperm fertilize an egg, and so the pregnancy miscarries.

Infections – a high temperature and some specific illnesses or infections, such as German measles, may cause miscarriage.

Anatomical problems – if the cervix (neck of the womb) is weak, it may start to open as the uterus becomes heavier in later pregnancy and this can lead to miscarriage, although this only accounts for 1 per cent of miscarriages.

Tests – Chorionic Villus Sampling (CVS) and amniocentesis, which are tests offered during some pregnancies, carry a 1–3 in 200 chance of miscarriage.

Radiation – the verdict is still out on whether or not radiation from visual display units (VDUs) can cause miscarriage, but enough concerns have been raised for you to at least limit the time you spend at the screen or to use a screen protector if you can.

Recovery time after miscarriage

How quickly you return to normal activities depends very much on the individual. You can expect to feel physically low for a week or so and you should try to take things easy during this time. We recommend that you do not attempt to return to work until you feel physically and emotionally strong, unless you find the routine, the support and sympathy of colleagues, and the focus of work, helpful.

Doctors' opinions vary on how long you should wait after a miscarriage before trying for another baby, and your fertility consultant will be able to advise you personally, but most recommend that you wait until you've had one period at the very least (which tends to be four to six weeks later). More importantly, you must feel physically and emotionally ready to try again. After a miscarriage, it is understandable to feel that you might never have a healthy baby. However, if you have conceived once, then you stand a good chance of getting pregnant again and the chances of having a successful pregnancy next time are better than you might think.

Where you are now

Congratulations. Let's savour the news that you are pregnant for a short while. After all, it's what you've been dreaming of for so long. You may find it hard, but relax and enjoy this pregnancy if you possibly can. Of course your emotions will be up and down and of course you will be concerned right up until you have a healthy baby in your arms, but don't lose sight of the fact that you have done a bold and difficult thing in getting this far and you should be justifiably proud of yourselves.

Perhaps you feel that you've reached the end of a long and hard journey but, in fact, you are at the start of a new one. As you set out, there will possibly be further ups and downs along the way, but it's important to know that there is help and support for you if you need it.

Even though I had a fantastic pregnancy and sailed through it and the birth, I never let myself think any further ahead than I was at the time. As a result, when Hema was born at 37 weeks, we had bought very few clothes and equipment.

Sarupa

After three cycles of Clomid, I couldn't believe I was pregnant. In fact, I didn't believe we would have Daniel right until the point that he was placed in my arms. I just felt there was so much that might go wrong and I felt that, with our luck, it was sure to happen to us.

Robyn

We had two unsuccessful IVF cycles and we'd decided that the third would be our last attempt. Just before I was due for my blood test, I got bad period pains and I was convinced it hadn't worked.

After the blood test, I got the call saying that it was a low positive and I should probably expect my period. The pains continued and I was just waiting for the period to start, but I got to the second blood test and still no period.

The results of the second test were much stronger and by the time it came to the scan, I could scarcely allow myself to hope, but there it was – a heartbeat and it was amazing.

Juliette

7

Sticking with it

In this chapter, we look at ways to sustain a positive approach and to keep moving forward when things seem to be going against you. Although receiving disappointing news is hard, try to hold on to the thought that there are:

- Strategies that will help you and your partner to cope with the immediate impact of negative results

- Actions that you can take to regain a sense of control and to help you make the right decisions for the future

- Tried and tested remedies for bolstering your emotional and physical well-being (which are invaluable now but will also last a lifetime).

We discuss all of the above in more detail in the following pages.

Receiving bad news

We know it can be tough going through fertility treatment and, sad to say, sometimes all your hard effort does not produce the results you long for. When a treatment does not work, it can be devastating. You are bound to feel sad, frustrated and upset, perhaps angry. **These feelings are natural and completely understandable and you have every right to feel as you do.**

If you can, it helps to express these feelings – try not to bottle them up. You may want to talk to friends and relatives, although many couples find that they can't face telling people about a negative result straightaway. In this case, why not consider talking to your fertility counsellor or to a support group? If you prefer, you can talk anonymously to a helpline (Infertility Network UK runs a helpline for members or you could try a general helpline such as the Samaritans – see Part 5 for details).

It can also be helpful to take some time to process your feelings before getting back into your normal routine. Perhaps you could take a break from work to look after yourself physically and emotionally. It is recommended that you give yourself time after such a disappointment to physically recover from the demands and stresses of treatment, but try to keep in the back of your mind that although this attempt did not work, it does not necessarily mean further treatments or a different method will not work for you in the future. You can talk to your specialist about the options when you feel the time is right.

Positive thinking

When we are knocked back by disappointments, it is common to feel that things will never go right, but negative thoughts can overwhelm us and turn a challenge into an insurmountable obstacle.

If possible, it is helpful at times of difficulty and disappointment to think positively. If you catch yourself thinking negative thoughts such as 'I'll never have a baby', then try turning that thought on its head into something positive such as 'I'm doing everything in my power to get pregnant.' Sounds too simple to be true, but it works.

In Eastern philosophies (and, increasingly, in the sporting arena), affirmations are used to bring positive outcomes and to challenge negative thinking. An affirmation involves stating out loud the way you would like things to be. So, for example, if your relationship is being adversely affected by the strain of a negative test result, you might stand in the shower saying, 'Everyday, in every way, we are getting stronger and closer.'

You can challenge your negative belief system and replace thoughts such as 'I don't deserve to be a parent' or that you're inadequate in some way with positive alternatives. You will be surprised at how your thoughts become more upbeat and you are more optimistic about the future.

If this all sounds a little airy-fairy to you, it's worth considering that research carried out in the US among a sample of women being treated for infertility showed that behavioural treatment, such as positive thinking techniques used to combat feelings of negativity, anxiety and depression, led to increased rates of conception.

Why didn't your treatment work?

You may experience feelings of failure and guilt after a negative test result and it's common to blame yourself but assisted reproductive technology (ART) is a complex and difficult process. There are various reasons why the procedure might not work – and none of them are you or your partner's fault, so please try not to blame yourselves. Although each case is individual, in general there are two stages at which things can go wrong. Initially, the treatment will not succeed if:

- your ovaries do not respond to the drugs used to stimulate egg production

- your ovaries over-respond (ovarian hyper-stimulation)

- no eggs are found at the egg collection stage

- your collected eggs don't fertilize (so there can be no embryos to transfer back to your womb)

- the embryos fail to develop in the laboratory.

Secondly, the most common reason why treatment does not work is if the embryo fails to grow in the womb. This could be for a number of reasons, including:

- low-quality embryos that do not mature or divide properly

- chromosomal problems with the embryos (new pre-implantation genetic screening – PGS – is reducing this problem)

- poor blood flow to the womb – even if the embryos are perfect, if blood flow to the uterus is poor, you have a lower chance of conceiving and a greater chance of miscarrying if you do get pregnant.

Getting more information

After a negative pregnancy test following fertility treatment, it is worth seeing your consultant, even if you're not sure whether you want to pursue further treatment.

There may be a lot you can learn about why the treatment didn't work and, depending at what stage of the process the treatment failed, there might be another option that can increase your chances of success if you choose to continue.

Is your relationship suffering?

Weathering the emotional turmoil of an unsuccessful treatment can bring you closer together as a couple. However, the emotional tension of undergoing fertility treatment, but especially when it's unsuccessful, can put a great strain on your relationship. Sometimes, such disappointments can cause us to retreat into our own worlds and this can cause problems in any loving relationship.

Good communication is at the heart of a good relationship and, if you are to come through this difficult time well, you and your partner should try to talk openly about your feelings, disappointments and hopes for the future. If you struggle to do this effectively, then the following tips, as recommended by Relate, the UK relationship-counselling organization may help:

• Set aside time to talk when you will not be interrupted.

• Take it in turns to have 'air time' – some people find setting a timer for five minutes, one speaking while the other listens, then reversing the process, can create a space for each to talk without interruption.

- Tell your partner how you feel about things without blaming them. This can be very tricky but it is a very useful way of being honest about how you feel.

- Plan to go somewhere that provides an environment you both find relaxing, for example, a walk in the park, a drink at a pub, or a coffee when you're shopping.

Don't be surprised if you don't see an instant improvement but, stick at it, and you will both see that things will get better between you.

If you are still having problems in your relationship, you could contact Relate, which has trained practitioners in the UK who can help you work through your problems. For your nearest Relate centre, go to **www.relate.org.uk** or call (local rates) 0845 456 1310 or 01788 573241.

Dealing with depression

It is natural to feel low when infertility treatment does not work or you have been trying for a long time without success. If your feelings of unhappiness are persistent and accompanied by a feeling of hopelessness you could be suffering from depression. Tick any of the following symptoms that apply to you:

❏ Poor appetite

❏ Sleeping difficulties

❏ Loss of energy

❏ Poor concentration

❏ Feelings of guilt

❏ Loss of interest in sex

❏ Shying away from activities previously enjoyed

❏ Fear of social gatherings

❏ Thoughts of death or suicide

Did you tick more than five? If so, you need expert and sympathetic help.

Getting help

If you suspect that you are suffering from depression and not a temporary 'low' as a natural reaction to continued difficulties in conceiving or to an unsuccessful treatment, you should consult your doctor or fertility counsellor straightaway. If you don't feel up to making an appointment, ask someone to do this for you or arrange for a home visit.

It is worth knowing that depression is readily treatable and most people get better either by a course of medication or by counselling, or both. Contrary to the myth, antidepressant drugs such as Prozac (fluoxetine) and Effexor (venlafaxine) are non-addictive. Occasionally, antidepressants interfere with hormone levels or lead to a loss of libido, so it is wise to tell your specialist about any drugs you are prescribed.

Often a short course of prescribed drugs will be followed by psychological support, and recovery takes place in almost every case. You are not being weak – depression is an illness and will-power alone cannot conquer disease. Rest assured that your symptoms will lift and this is where the depression helplines (see Part 5, page 314) can be hugely beneficial. These helplines are frequently staffed by people who have had depression themselves and they know what you're going through.

Hard though it may be, the most important thing you can do for yourself is to believe that you *will* get better and to be patient – your recovery may take a little while. There are also several precautions you can take to hasten the recovery process:

- Get as much rest as you can. Tiredness aggravates depression so try to have adequate sleep and rest.

- You must eat sensibly and regularly. Low blood sugar levels (hypoglycaemia) can make you feel even more wretched. Sometimes, vitamin B6, a multi-mineral or a general vitamin supplement is recommended.

- Try to keep things in proportion. Yes, fertility treatment is stressful, but you can cope.

- Be kind to yourself – avoid commitments that give you anxiety and concentrate on busying yourself with things that you enjoy.

Moving on

Only you and your partner will know when the time is right to make a decision about whether to have another attempt with your existing treatment or whether to look at other alternatives.

After a failed treatment, some women are keen to try again almost straightaway. It's as if they want to put this result behind them and move on. For other women, a break from treatment to give the body a chance to recover, to take stock and to process emotions makes more sense. Sometimes couples give themselves three to six months' rest and then resume treatment – understandably, this option may not be appropriate for older women. Others feel that they cannot go through the process again and they wish to consider other options.

When you're feeling knocked back by a failed treatment, it can be heartening to know that there are couples who have a successful pregnancy after numerous attempts at ART, and you often hear that a couple were about to give up treatment when they finally conceived.

However, there is no wrong or right choice about whether to continue with treatment or not, just the one that is right for you. Whatever your feelings – and remember, nothing is written in stone, you can always change your mind at a later date and resume treatment when you feel ready – it is worth speaking with your specialist to get his or her advice so that you can take this into account when coming to a decision.

Considering other treatments

It is possible that the treatment(s) you have undergone so far, for various reasons, are no longer recommended or viable for you. Although this is not the news you want to hear, it doesn't mean that you have exhausted all routes to having a baby. Having exhausted standard ART, depending on your circumstances and the causes for your inability to conceive, your specialist might recommend ART using donated sperm, eggs or embryos.

Donor Conception

How do you know it's right for you?

There are certain circumstances, which we explain in greater detail below, but in brief, where if you have no ovaries or are producing very few if any eggs, or if your partner is producing little or no sperm, for example, then using donated sperm, eggs or embryos can be the most appropriate route for you to have a baby.

In fact, nearly 2,000 babies are born every year in the UK using donated sperm, eggs or embryos but it is not a treatment to undertake without careful consideration. You and your partner will have to discuss how you feel about one or possibly both of you having no genetic connection with your baby. You may still be coming to terms with the fact that other fertility treatment has been unsuccessful, and you should give yourselves time to adjust to this new approach and to think it through thoroughly before committing to treatment. You won't be pressurized into making a decision and you should take your time, only going ahead if you both feel ready. Things you might like to discuss and consider include:

- How do you feel about using eggs, sperm or embryos from someone you don't know?

- How important is genetic connection to you?

- Will you feel jealous if a donor conceives a child with your partner?

- How will it affect your relationship with your respective families?

- Will you tell your child about the way they were conceived?

- How will you feel if your child decides to contact the donor when they are 18?

- Is it better to use a donor unknown to you or to find your own donor?

- How do you feel about your child or children sharing a partial genetic link with children in other families? (A donor's sperm can be used to create up to ten families excluding their own.)

Most clinics run local patient support groups and the UK Donor Conception Network (see Part 5, page 303) is a national support network for people considering treatment using donor eggs, sperm or embryos. Both are there to help you in your deliberations and it can be very useful to talk to other couples who have been through the same decision process that you are going through.

However, when considering the pros and cons of such a decision it is worth bearing in mind that genetic connection is not what makes a loving family. Many parents who have a child or children using donated eggs, sperm or embryos say that the joy of becoming a family more than compensates for lack of genetic connection.

Using donated sperm

This technique is also known as donor insemination (DI) and it is recommended in cases where:

- your partner is producing little or no sperm

- your partner's sperm is unlikely to be able to fertilize an egg

- your partner has a risk of passing on an inherited disease

- your partner has had a vasectomy that cannot be reversed.

After checks to make sure you are producing eggs and that your fallopian tubes are healthy (you may also be offered fertility drugs to optimize your chances), treatment will be arranged to coincide with your ovulation. The donor sperm are introduced into the neck of your womb (cervix) or the womb itself using a thin tube (see intrauterine insemination – IUI – page 116). Your partner may well be allowed to be with you during the procedure.

Since you are using your own eggs in this procedure, the chances of success are greatly affected by your age. If you're under 35, the success rate is around 14 per cent for each attempt. This falls to 8–9 per cent if you're between 35–39 years old and 4-5 per cent if you're between 40 and 42.

If you would like to have more than one child, provided the sperm is available and the donor's consent permits, you could use the same donor so that your children will be full genetic siblings. In this case, before your first attempt, it is worth letting your clinic know that you may wish to use the same donor in the future.

Q. I am in a long-term lesbian relationship and we would like to have a baby using donated sperm. Is this possible?

A. Clinics vary in their eligibility criteria. Some offer donor insemination to single and lesbian women and it is worth checking with your chosen clinic at the outset. By law, before agreeing to treatment, a clinic must consider your potential baby's welfare and that includes 'the need for a father'. As such, we would expect that you might be asked about your plans for raising a child in a lesbian relationship, just as a single mother would be asked about her plans for raising a child alone.

Using donated eggs

This involves another woman donating her egg(s), which are then fertilized in a laboratory by your partner's or donor sperm. The resulting embryo is then placed in your uterus, as in standard IVF (see page 117) and you'll be given hormonal drugs in order to maintain the pregnancy. Occasionally, the sperm and eggs are introduced together into the uterus before fertilization takes place (Gamete Intra-Fallopian Transfer – GIFT – see page 125). You might consider egg donation as a route to having a baby if:

- you are producing few or low quality eggs

- you have no ovaries or have had them removed

- you are post-menopausal

- you have had cancer treatment that has damaged your ovaries

- you have a hormonal imbalance

- you have had recurrent miscarriages

- you have tried to conceive unsuccessfully using fertility drugs or IVF

- you have a high risk of passing on a serious inherited genetic disorder.

There is a good success rate for using donor eggs – on average 25–40 per cent per treatment – which is slightly higher than the average success rate for conventional IVF across all age groups because donor eggs must come from someone aged 35 or younger. However, the waiting list for donor eggs in the UK is long (around two years) and, in light of the latest legal changes to donor anonymity, set to get longer. If you feel time is against you, you might wish to ask suitable friends or relatives to donate, or speak to your clinic because some women receiving treatment are prepared to donate eggs if enough are collected and they have some spare. You could also advertise for a donor. In March 2007, Richard and Linda Weeks of Maidstone, England took out an ad campaign on the inside of 50 buses. After years of fertility treatment, their only hope of having their own baby was through egg donation, so they were delighted to receive more than 60 responses – the story made the national newspapers where it captured the hearts and minds of the nation.

Another alternative in the UK is to use donated eggs from abroad, where the supply is more plentiful because donors are paid. However, there are drawbacks. Imported eggs from abroad must satisfy Human Fertilisation and Embryology Authority (HFEA) standards, i.e. donor screening etc., and they must have been obtained under conditions comparable to those in the UK. Moreover, if you seek treatment abroad, clinics are not regulated by the HFEA code and so you must satisfy yourself about the standard of treatment you can expect from any clinic you are considering. You should ask about donor selection practices and the rights to information about the donor for you and any child born from the donation. Bear in mind that in the UK, the egg donor has no legal responsibility or rights in respect of children born as a result of their donation – this is not always the case in other countries, so you would need to seek independent legal advice and you should not rely on the assurances of the clinic alone.

Q. We are using donated eggs. If we have a child, will I be its legal mother?

A. By law, the woman receiving the treatment is the baby's mother, not the woman who donated the eggs. When your partner gave his consent to the treatment, by law, he became the baby's legal father.

Using donated embryos

This form of treatment may be an option for you if:

- you and/or your partner have fertility problems that are likely to prevent other treatment that uses your own sperm and/or eggs from being successful

- you and your partner are both at high risk of passing on serious inheritable conditions

- you are single and post-menopausal.

This procedure is exactly the same as if you were undergoing standard IVF with frozen embryos (see Chapter 4, page 117), except that the embryos are donated rather than your own. Wherever possible, the clinic will use donated embryos from donors whose characteristics closely match those of you and your partner. Most donated embryos are from couples who have completed their treatment (either successfully and their family is complete, or they have chosen to discontinue treatment), or some couples donate surplus embryos that they cannot use in their own treatment which they do not wish to freeze.

Q. If we use a donated embryo, what are the chances that the baby will look like me or my partner?

A. Every effort is made to match donor and patient characteristics so there's a good chance that your child will resemble you or your partner. However, just as with naturally conceived children, there's an outside chance that the child will not look like you, your husband or the donor. There is a shortage of eggs, sperm and embryos from some ethnic groups so if you wish to receive from a donor from such a group, you may want to consider finding your own donor.

Donor identification

Until April 2005 in the UK, if you conceived using donated sperm, eggs or embryos, the donor could remain anonymous. However, the law in the UK has now changed. As a result, all children born from donated sperm, eggs and embryos will be entitled to certain **non-identifying** information about their donor once they reach the age of 18. This information includes:

- physical characteristics such as height and colouring

- year and country of birth

- ethnic group (and that of his/her parents)

- whether they were adopted

- marital status

- gender and number of children they already have (if applicable)

- details of donor screening tests and medical history

- any other information the donor provided at the time of donation.

If the donor registered (or re-registered) after 1 April 2005, the following identifying information will also be made available to donor-conceived children, on request, once they are 18:

- name, and name at birth if different

- date and place of birth

- latest known address

- physical appearance

- donor ID number at the centre.

In effect, this means that your donor-conceived child could decide to contact that donor when they come of age. Of course, your child might not be interested in knowing anything about that person, let alone meeting them, but it is important to give some thought as to how this might affect you because it is a possibility.

For more information on what information can be given to a donor-conceived person, their parents and to the donor and about the Donor Register in the UK, visit **www.hfea.gov.uk**.

Q. We have a beautiful six-month old baby girl after using donated eggs to conceive. My husband and I can't agree about if and when we should tell her that I am not her genetic mother. What if she finds it shocking?

A. Knowing the right time to tell your daughter about the way she was conceived will not be easy but it is crucial that she learns about her origins from you rather than anyone else. Perhaps when she is at the age where children ask the inevitable questions about where babies come from, for example, it would be a good time to introduce the idea. When she's older, you could give her more details, if she wants to know.

If you talk openly and naturally about her conception, there is no reason why she should feel any different from any other child. The Donor Conception Network offers support and advice to parents of donor-conceived children and they have literature to help you to tell children about donor conception (see Part 5, Chapter 12, page 303).

So much to take in

As you can see, donor conception is a complex concept that can provoke unexpected and conflicting emotions and reactions in people. At this point, it's worth pausing for thought and, at your own pace, re-reading the information we have given you. It is something that you and your partner will need to discuss as candidly and openly as possible and you should try to be sensitive to the other's feelings, which may differ from your own.

As it is such a complex issue, we strongly recommend that you do not come to a decision without seeking some additional advice. Perhaps talk to your clinic's own counsellor, your specialist, a support network such as the Donor Conception Network , online support groups or an experienced counsellor.

What about surrogacy?

If you are unable to carry a baby to term or are unable to conceive in any medically assisted way, asking someone else to have a baby for you may be your only remaining option, but this is a route to parenthood that involves a high degree of commitment by you, your partner and the surrogate mother. There are two main categories of surrogacy:

1 You and your partner can use your own egg and sperm to create an embryo, which is implanted in the womb of the surrogate mother at a clinic (known as 'partial surrogacy' or sometimes 'gestational' or 'host IVF surrogacy').

2 If your eggs are not suitable, you can use your partner's sperm to artificially fertilize the surrogate mother's own eggs (known as 'full surrogacy' or sometimes 'traditional' or 'straight surrogacy').

The second option is medically more straightforward because it can take place using a simple kit provided by the surrogacy agency without any involvement from health professionals. However, if you can produce viable embryos, many couples opt to try clinic-assisted partial surrogacy (your own eggs and sperm). Despite the much higher outlay incurred by IVF costs, this can give them their own baby rather than a baby who is only biologically related to the male partner.

The cost of surrogacy

If you are using clinic surrogacy that involves ART treatment, then it can cost over £25,000 including around £10,000 that is usually paid to the surrogate to compensate her for clothing, travel expenses, loss of earning, etc. Quite apart from the financial consideration, surrogacy can also be costly emotionally. Those who have been through it recommend that you enlist the support of friends, family and surrogacy support networks.

Where would you start?

As with the other treatments that we've discussed in this chapter, the surrogacy process is one that requires a great deal of consideration before starting out. Perhaps more than any other assisted route to parenthood, surrogacy involves moral, emotional and legal implications that may affect you, your partner and your child not just now but in the future. Consequently, it is very important that you seek advice from an experienced counsellor as your first port of call and, at some point before starting out, you will need to get legal advice too.

MYTH: If a surrogate mother carries and gives birth to your child, you will not bond with your baby.

FACT: You do not have to be genetically connected to your baby to feel love and connection. The parent–child bond develops through everyday caring and spending time with your baby – soothing her, bathing her, cuddling and playing with her. As you spend more and more time in eye contact with your baby and holding her – skin to skin contact (holding her against your own skin) whenever possible is excellent – so your bond will build and grow. We're sure you will have no problems in falling in love with your baby and she will love you and your partner in return.

If you are going to use your own eggs and your partner's sperm, your licensed IVF clinic will have a counsellor who can talk through some of the implications of what is involved. Alternatively, you could speak to one of the advisers at a surrogacy agency such as Childlessness Overcome Through Surrogacy (COTS) or Surrogacy UK who are well versed in all the legal and emotional aspects of the surrogacy process (see Part 5 for further details).

How do you find a surrogate?

Perhaps you have a relative or friend who is willing to help you to achieve your dream of having a baby, or you may prefer to find a surrogate that you don't already know. It is illegal for a fertility clinic to find a surrogate for you but an agency like COTS has a register of about three surrogates to every five couples who approach them. Happily, some surrogates are prepared to have more than one baby, so most couples have a chance to at least try surrogacy with one surrogate.

It's worth talking to other people who have experienced surrogacy to find out how they found their surrogate but, by law, you are not allowed to advertise for a surrogate. If you go through an agency, you will be matched with a surrogate and given time to get to know each other before any agreement is made. It's very important that you get on and that you agree on issues that might affect you or the pregnancy, such as antenatal testing, for example. Everyone who has been through the process stresses the importance of absolute trust.

Should you decide to go ahead, you'll be offered ongoing support, advice and guidance by qualified, experienced staff along with help on the legal processes (see below) when the baby is born. The agency is also there to mediate in the event of a disagreement between you as a couple and your surrogate. Thankfully, such disagreements are rare and 99.5 per cent of surrogacies in the UK are concluded satisfactorily.

What the law says about surrogacy

Surrogacy agencies can advise you and help you with the legal requirements of surrogacy or you can seek advice from a solicitor before making any decisions. However, in brief, here are the main legal points that you should be aware of:

- **As the woman giving birth, the surrogate is the legal mother of the child at birth.** Her name will be put on the birth certificate until you have applied through the courts for a parental order or adoption. Legal parentage is then transferred to you, or to you and your partner as a couple.

- **Usually, the surrogate's partner or husband is the legal father at birth.** His name will appear on the birth certificate until you apply through the courts for a parental order or to adopt the child. In Scotland, it's possible for your partner's name to appear on the birth certificate, giving him legal parentage.

- **The surrogate mother has the legal right to change her mind, even if the baby is not genetically related to her.** This happens very rarely but this is why it is so essential that you trust each other and are clear and committed to your arrangement from the outset.

- **It is illegal to pay a surrogate in the UK.** You can pay 'reasonable expenses' such as costs incurred by the surrogate for clothes, travel expenses and loss of earnings, etc.

- **You can only apply for a parental order if you and your partner are married, living in the UK and if the child is genetically related to either one or both of you.** To apply for a parental order, the surrogate and the father of the child must agree unconditionally to this being made, and the order must be applied for within six months of the birth. Legal advice should be sought.

- **If you do not qualify for a parental order, you must adopt the child.** Your clinic is breaking the law if they provide treatment before ascertaining that a registered adoption agency is involved in the process. Again, legal advice should be sought.

I decided to donate my eggs because I loved being pregnant and I wanted to help women who couldn't experience it on their own to have a chance to go through it too.

I often wonder if it worked. I donated nearly two dozen eggs and am curious to know if the eggs were good enough quality to help someone, but I'm not tempted to find out myself.

I wonder if one day someone will knock on the door and tell me they are my egg! I am not scared about this, a little bit curious but that's all. My family know I donated – I couldn't have done it without the help of my partner (he injected me daily!!!) – and my children occasionally wonder if they have another half-sibling on the planet.

Liz

After seeing a television programme in 1994 on surrogacy, with her family's support, Carol decided to become a surrogate. She was 23 years old when she became a surrogate for the first time.

My third surrogacy was for a wonderful couple that I had known for about a year and I had been following their story. Pip had been born without a womb so never had the chance of even trying for a baby. I was their third surrogate. The first tried for about two years but did not fall pregnant, unfortunately. The second fell pregnant but miscarried at around ten weeks. My heart went out to them so I offered to be their surrogate.

Our first try at insemination was unsuccessful. But after the second, I phoned them up as giddy as a school child to tell them I was pregnant.

In the early hours of the morning on 15 August, the contractions started to get strong, so Dermott, my husband, phoned Pip and Kevin. Pip's mum stayed at my house to look after my kids and the four of us went to the hospital.

At 7:55 a.m. Baby Kitty was born straight into Pip's hands. She weighed 7lb 14oz and was gorgeous. Kevin tried to cut the cord but said he couldn't see it for the tears of joy in his eyes (he nearly cut the midwife's finger's instead), but he managed in the end.

After a while Pip, Kevin and their daughter Kitty were taken to a room next door to spend some precious time alone. It was lovely seeing them all together and seeing how happy they are.

We stayed in touch and, because of this, I knew how much they wanted a sibling, so I offered to carry a second child for them. Archie was born on Easter Monday 2005.

I would like to thank my husband Dermott and my three children as without their help and support I could never have accomplished what I have.

Carol

For Carol's full story plus those of other surrogate mothers, go to **www.surrogacyuk.org**

8

Life beyond treatment

As you have seen, there are many different issues that affect whether or not you can have a baby, and equally there are many varying factors that influence the choices you make in achieving that goal. At the start of this book, you might have said that you and your partner wanted a baby at any price. However, after all that you've read, or perhaps after a series of unsuccessful attempts at infertility treatment, you may have decided that there are limits to what you are prepared to undergo.

Some couples decide from the outset that medical intervention is not an option that is right for them, and they continue to leave getting pregnant or otherwise in the hands of Nature. Some couples undergo treatment but reach a point where they decide that, financially, physically or emotionally, they cannot afford more treatment. For others, the decision to stop is prompted by news from their doctor that they have exhausted treatment options, while some simply feel they have given it their best shot and that they now want to get on with life.

Moving on

Although your desire for a child may remain undiminished, you may nonetheless come to a point where, for whatever reason, you decide that enough is enough. Sometimes, recognizing that you want to stop treatment can come as a sudden bolt from the blue and sometimes it is a more gradual realization but, although it is difficult, it is important that you feel you are making a choice to stop. If not, it may feel as if you have failed or not done enough, although this is simply not the case and you should not torment yourself.

Of course, deciding to stop treatment does not mean that you have to give up all hope of having children – you may wish to explore the possibility of adoption or fostering, which we discuss in more detail later in this chapter (see pages 242 and 246).

Deciding to end treatment can be a painful process and both you and your partner must talk it through and agree that the time is right to stop. At this stage, it is often helpful to talk to a counsellor, or to others who have been through a similar decision process as you start to think about moving on. (See information on the organization More to Life, page 305).

Deciding to stop treatment

If you think the time may be right to stop treatment but you are not sure, there are some questions that you and your partner might like to think about, and the answers may help to crystallize your feelings:

	Yes	No
Are you continuing with treatment to avoid disappointing someone else such as your partner, or even your doctor/clinic?	❏	❏
Do you feel you have tried every available avenue?	❏	❏
Do you still feel excited when you consider treatment plans or do you resent it?	❏	❏
Is it more important to you to be pregnant or to be a parent?	❏	❏
Have you thought about other family-building options?	❏	❏

                                                Yes No

Is the dream of having your
own biological child dimming?   ❏   ❏

- How would you feel if your doctor told
  you that there was nothing more that
  could be done?

- How far are you prepared to allow
  technology enter into conceiving a
  child?

Your reactions to some of these questions
may surprise you. If you can both give
some consideration to these issues and
discuss them candidly, the answers may
help you and your partner come to a
decision that feels right for you both,
whether that means giving it another try,
having a break or stopping treatment.

Q. Giving up on our dream of having our own baby after so much investment and struggle seems unthinkable but we're so tired of treatment. Should we stop?

A. If you are undecided, you might like to consider taking a break from treatment. If you then reassess how you feel after, say, six months, you may have a clearer idea of how much further you're prepared to go. Conversely, the sense of relief at having your lives back during 'the break' may be enough to help you to decide to stop treatment altogether. A break can be a good compromise for weary couples.

Dealing with how you are feeling

Although giving up on your dream of having a baby yourself is undoubtedly difficult, making an active decision can also bring a sense of resolution, and perhaps surprisingly, this is often accompanied by a feeling of accomplishment.

Having come through the physical and emotional challenges of fertility treatment, many couples report that they feel they can conquer anything in life together. Surviving the experience of tests, investigations and treatment and the emotional highs and lows can give some couples a renewed self-esteem and confidence.

However, initially, as you come to terms with the implications of your decision to stop treatment and as you work towards that resolution, you may feel:

- exhausted and drained, physically and emotionally

- grief for the baby you won't have

- a sense of loss – as the routine of medical treatment ends, so too does the hope of what treatment might bring

- anger and a strong sense of injustice

- frightened about what the future holds.

These painful emotions may be tempered by the conflicting feelings of:

- relief that you won't have to go through the emotional roller-coaster and physical challenge again

- pride that you have survived such a difficult process

- having a greater closeness with your partner

- acceptance that you cannot change or completely control every aspect of your life

- optimism for a bright future without the anxiety of trying for a baby.

This range of conflicting emotions is perfectly natural, and how you feel is likely to change from day to day. It can take some time for these feelings to settle down and for you to feel that you really are able to move on. Again, this is normal and understandable, and you shouldn't feel you have to rush. Similarly, you don't have to tell friends and family of your decision until you are ready. As you move towards feeling comfortable with your decision, the following coping strategies may help.

Coping strategies

- Seek emotional support and guidance from friends, relatives, a counsellor or support group.

- Talk with others who have successfully found different paths after infertility.

- Invest time and energy in your relationship.

- Be kind to yourselves and take as much time and space as it takes to fully recover.

- Remind yourselves regularly that you are a valuable person in your own right whether you have children or not.

- Pursue hobbies and activities that you and your partner can do together.

- Re-establish contact with friends and family with whom you may have lost touch during treatment.

- Have a holiday that you could not contemplate if you were pregnant or had a baby with you.

- Make plans for the future, if that helps.

Next steps: adoption and fostering

The fertility treatments discussed in Chapters 4 and 7 are not the only way to help you to have a family. You may wish to explore the options of adoption or fostering. These are not easy or instant solutions and they are not right for everyone, but you may want to take these alternative routes to parenthood into account when deciding the best way to move forward.

Q. What's the difference between adoption and fostering?

A. Adoptive parents have full parental responsibility for a child whereas foster carers share the responsibility for the child with a local authority and the child's parents. Fostering is usually temporary while adoption is a permanent arrangement.

MYTH: You have to be young and married to adopt a child.

FACT: In fact, there is no upper age limit for adoption and single people as well as those in homosexual relationships may be eligible to adopt. There are in fact very few restrictions on who can adopt (a certain type of criminal record may be an obstacle, for example – see **www.baaf.org.uk** or call the Adoption UK helpline on 0844 848 7900 for fuller details of who is eligible). The main criteria for eligibility are that you have to be over 21, happy to make space in your life and home for a child, patient, flexible and energetic, and determined to make a real difference to a child's life, for a lifetime.

Adoption

The path from undergoing fertility treatment to admitting infertility to pursuing adoption involves many difficult questions, none of which have hard and fast right answers. Yet, for many couples, adoption is a good and responsible way to become parents.

Adoption is a legal procedure under which the child you have adopted becomes part of your family. It legally removes the rights and responsibilities of the child's birth parent(s), and transfers them to you. The child will take your surname and, once an adoption order has been granted, it cannot be reversed (except in very rare cases).

MYTH: You will conceive as soon as you adopt a child.

FACT: Although there is some truth in the idea that when a couple adopts a child the pressure of 'trying for a baby' is off and they do go on to get pregnant, in fact, the conception rate stays the same (about 5 per cent) as those couples with fertility problems who do not adopt. Adopting a child can be wonderful but it should not be viewed as a route to pregnancy.

How would you go about adoption?

There are up to 4,000 children in the UK waiting for new families. If you think you might like to try to adopt a child, the first step is to contact an adoption agency. Some agencies – like Barnardo's – are voluntary societies, but the majority are part of the local authority children's services (in England and Wales) or social work (in Scotland) department. You can find an agency near you on the British Association for Adoption and Fostering (BAAF) agency database (see Part 5, Chapter 12) or your local authority's contact details will be in your phone book. Once you contact an agency, they will send you detailed literature on how adoption works and the process you would go through should you decide to go ahead.

How do you find a child?

It usually takes at least six months for social workers from an adoption agency to get to know you, to assess you and to help you to prepare for a future with an adopted family. Once approved, the agency will try to match you with a suitable child or children (over half of all children waiting for adoption are in groups of brothers and sisters who need to be placed together).

If the proposed match is approved – and it's worth pointing out that the process focuses on the needs of the child and matching them to the right parents, not on the needs of the prospective

---

MYTH: There are no babies for adoption in the UK.

FACT: There are children waiting for new families of all ages, ethnicity and religious backgrounds. Young babies are rarer than infants and school-aged children, and you may have to wait for some time if you want to adopt a baby. As a result, some couples decide to adopt from overseas where there are more babies needing adoptive families.

There are agencies and local authorities who have specialist knowledge of inter-country adoption and the BAAF also has literature on the subject (see Part 5, Chapter 12).

Any adoption is a significant step to take for you and the child, but adopting a child from a different race and culture can involve even more complex issues, so it needs very careful consideration. There are also financial implications to take into account in adopting from another country (costs vary depending on the country) whereas adoption within the UK does not involve any financial expenditure, apart from the normal costs of having a child.

parents – then, after a period of introductions and meetings, the child will move in to live with you. But, don't worry, you won't be left completely alone to fend for yourselves. Social workers will remain involved to support you and your new family for as long as you feel is necessary and there are support groups run by many of the voluntary organizations where adoptive parents can swap advice and experiences.

After a certain minimum period of living together as a family, an application can be submitted for the adoption to be made legal in court.

Q. Can we start adoption procedures if we are still actively trying to conceive through fertility treatment?

A. Most adoption agencies would caution against starting adoption procedures if you are still involved in treatment. The received wisdom is that you should exhaust all infertility treatment avenues or make a conscious decision to stop treatment and give yourselves time to come to terms with that decision before actively pursuing the adoption route.

Nonetheless, you can certainly research the adoption option while still trying to conceive.

Fostering

The aim of fostering is to provide a family for children who cannot live with their own parents. It is usually a temporary arrangement while the child's parents get help sorting out their problems or take a break, or it helps children through a difficult period in their lives. The children then return home once the problems that caused them to come into foster care have been resolved.

Since the aim of successful fostering is to provide a happy short-term solution, not to create a family, fostering can be a challenging option for couples who originally wanted to be parents.

Undoubtedly, there can be great rewards in being able to offer a child help through a tricky time by bringing him or her into your home. However, it can also be emotionally demanding and it can be difficult to know that the child will eventually leave and return to his or her own family.

What do you need to do to be a foster carer?

If you are interested in becoming a foster carer, the first step is to get in touch with your local authority's fostering team or with a fostering agency in your area. You can find details in the phone book or in the BAAF agency database (see Part 5, Chapter 12).

You and your partner will need to go through thorough preparation and assessment to become foster carers. You will receive training and visits from a social worker and, once you are approved as a foster carer, there are annual reviews and continued training.

Q. Is it true that foster carers get paid?

A. All foster carers receive an allowance to cover the cost of caring for a child in their home, and there are certain tax and national insurance incentives for foster carers, but they are not paid as such. However, increasingly, fostering is being considered as a 'professional' role and many local authorities, voluntary and independent fostering agencies run schemes to pay foster carers a fee that is linked to a child's particular needs and is sometimes a reflection of the skills, ability and length of experience a foster carer has.

Staying as a couple

Adoption and fostering are not the right options for everyone and so it may be that after a decision to stop treatment or if getting pregnant is simply not happening for you, you prefer to stay as a couple and explore what life without children has to offer.

Although it is hard to give up on your dreams of parenthood, it is important that you and your partner come to an active decision to move on to another chapter of life whether you have had unsuccessful treatment or have never had treatment. Making a choice to get on with living rather than feeling that your life is on hold can help you to feel a greater sense of control, purpose and direction.

It would be trite to say that such a decision will not be without sadness, but perhaps stepping off the infertility treadmill may, with time, give you an opportunity to appreciate the good things you have in your life and to plan for a bright future. Your decision will probably cause you to rethink what you expected from life and reassess what you now wish to achieve, and this can be both painful as well as an opportunity for excitement and optimism.

Only those who have personal experience of what you're going through can really understand what it is like, but try not to feel isolated or alone. There are many other couples who have had similar experiences to what you are going through now. If you want to share your thoughts and feelings with others who have been through it, there is a national network, More to Life (part of Infertility Network UK), which is dedicated solely to providing a support service to those who, involuntarily, will remain without children. They can offer support to help you to adjust to this new time in your lives and, if necessary, to grieve for what might have been. More to Life has a lending library of useful books and factsheets, a daytime telephone advice line (08701 188088) and a network of members through the UK (see Part 5, Chapter 12).

Alternatively, counselling might help – you could either speak to an infertility counsellor through your clinic or contact the British Association for Counselling and Psychotherapy (BACP) on 0870 443 5252 for a list of local counsellors (see Part 5, Chapter 12). If you want to speak to someone without delay and in confidence, call Careline, the national telephone counselling service on 0845 122 8622.

Initially, while the decision to live life without children is raw, you may not feel optimistic about the future, but couples who have made the same decision as you and who are further down the road can tell you that there are plenty of positive and fulfilling ways to have a good life and to enjoy each other's company to the full. Try to hold on to the thought that you do not have to be parents to be a valuable person and to lead a rewarding life.

Little by little, as you come to terms with your disappointment, you may find that a childfree lifestyle has lots to recommend it. Some of the benefits that couples report include:

- freedom to make decisions without having to worry about how it might affect others (within reason)

- time to think things through and not having to spend your life in a rush

- spontaneity – being able to take off for the weekend or to make last-minute changes to plans

- a chance to follow hobbies and holidays that are not child-friendly

- being cash-rich so you can make the odd impulse buy without having to think too much about it

- the opportunity to think about what you might want for the future

- time for yourself so you can treat yourself to a massage or a lie-in at the weekend.

It may not seem possible at the moment, but there will come a time when you are able to enjoy life to the full again, and you can plan for a happy future.

In January 2002, Helen and her partner were given the heartbreaking news that he had a virtually non-existent sperm count with low motility. They tried ICSI (intra-cytoplasmic sperm injction) treatment six times in all – four fresh cycles and two frozen – but were unsuccessful.

> *In spite of all the unanswered questions and years of dashed hopes, we have been able to put this behind us and have moved on to a much happier place. I still want to be a mum and with God's help I believe I will be. For me it isn't about giving birth, it's about being a parent and I am delighted to be able to tell you that we were approved to become adoptive parents in April 2006.*
>
> *I stopped treatment at the age of 35 because I knew I didn't want to lose out on the relatively young years of motherhood that I knew I could definitely have with adoption. Believe me, once you take the first nervous steps into the adoption community, there is a world of support and endless, wonderful, uplifting stories of people's experiences and normal family lives;*

*news of which my husband and I have
been in such need of for years.*

*So if you are feeling broken with
grief, the way I did for so long, then
please take heart and believe you are a
valuable person with a life worth living,
for others as well as yourself. I hope our
story has helped someone feel a little
better.*

*You may wish to continue with
fertility treatment, I personally felt the
need to keep on trying for as long as I
did, but knew when it was time to stop.
You may become pregnant or you may
not, but if like me you don't, this does
not mean the end to your dreams of
becoming a parent. There are so many
children out there in need of a loving
and secure home and we are really
excited about becoming a mum and dad.*

Helen

Coping strategies

If you are just adjusting to the idea of planning a life that does not feature your own children, these strategies may help:

- Try to think positively. Hope and excitement about the future and discussing your new plans with your partner can help.

- Bolster each other's self-esteem. Your value as a person is not measured in your ability to have a baby.

- Spend time with people who make you feel good and uplifted.

- Enjoy your work – get your teeth into a new project or, alternatively, ask about a sabbatical to travel or to invest time in a hobby or pursuit you enjoy.

- Exercise. Getting fresh air and plenty of exercise releases the body's natural endorphins (mood-lifters) and helps to combat negative thoughts.

Part 4:
Real Lives

9

Your letters

In this part of the book you will find typical stories of couples facing various fertility issues. Reading stories of others who have been through similar experiences to your own can be a real comfort. Being alone with your problems is very hard, and it helps to know that someone else has been there too.

This part will not only help you to see that you are not alone, but it will also show you that infertility can affect anyone, irrespective of age, background or gender. This chapter has letters from the postbag – a series of questions and answers, and Chaper 10 details your stories of fertility issues and treatment. We hope that the following stories will help you to see that, with the right help and loving support, you can hopefully achieve your goal of having a baby and move on to happier times.

From the postbag

Letters to *This Morning* are never disclosed to anyone but these created letters are typical of the hundreds received each week.

Dear Denise,

I'm in my second round of IVF and I'm terrified it won't work. Apart from that, I feel my partner is going off the idea of our ever having a family of our own. He keeps pointing out that his sister and her husband never have a holiday and live in a pokey little house with their three children. I know he's hinting that could be us if we go ahead, especially when the IVF is costing us money we don't have. I find myself getting very resentful of his attitude because he was the one who went on about having kids in the first place. Half of me wants to just pull out and say to hell with it all. The other half of me says a life without children would be no life at all. I feel as though I'm damned if it happens and damned if it doesn't. At this rate I may not even have a relationship at the end of it all.

Dear X,

My guess is that your husband is scared of
failure and is trying to cushion the blow for
you by pointing out there are snags as well
as bonuses in having a family. He's doing
this because he loves you to bits and can't
bear to see you unhappy. Give him a big
cuddle and tell him how you feel. That will
give him a chance to tell you how he feels
and together you can decide whether or not
going ahead is worth it. Of course it can be
expensive and time-consuming and
frustrating and you have to be very sure it's
what you really want to do. If it is, the
rewards can be great. If you can, plan an
evening out and talk it through when you're
both relaxed. If you want to blow off steam
in the meantime, Careline in the UK (Tel:
0845 122 8622) will lend a listening ear to
anyone who needs to offload pain and
anxiety so that they can carry on towards
their goal.

Dear Denise,
The only way I can afford IVF is to trade my
eggs but I have severe worries about this. How
am I going to feel knowing there are children
growing up somewhere who are mine and I'll
never know them. What if those eggs work and
my own embryos fail? Someone else will have
my children and I'll have none. And I worry
too...so does my mother...that one day two of
my children could meet up and never know they
were sister and brother. With all these things to
worry about, how can I go ahead with it? And
yet if I don't, I can't afford the treatment. It just
seems like there's no way out.

Dear X,

These questions are quite understandable
and have been voiced to me many times
before. Yes, there will be children created
from your eggs but they will have been
carried in the womb by another woman and
fertilized by her husband so they won't be
the same as the child you and your partner
make together and which you carry for nine
months before you give birth. There is a risk
that that the other woman's pregnancy

might be successful and yours not, but the alternative is that you don't go forward and will be left childless anyway.

As for the risk of children meeting, in the huge pool of people in the UK, that is unlikely, but you are entitled to question the doctors about where the eggs will be donated and ask that it be in another part of the country. That doesn't rule out a meeting but makes it a little less likely.

Infertility Network, the national infertility support network, can be contacted on 08701 188088 and will provide you with information and support. They'll have heard the questions you ask many times before and will understand your need for answers. Decisions must be made by you and your partner, but find out all you can before you let your chance of a child slip away. Remember, too, that you have the opportunity to bring enormous happiness to another couple who are facing a childless future.

Dear Denise,

I've been through all the tests and my gynaecologist tells me there is no reason why I can't have children. He wants my husband to be tested but he won't. It's his mother who is stopping it. She says he's always been healthy and it can't possibly be him at fault. I know she blames me. Her daughter, my sister-in-law, has four children and she's always going on about them and making me feel a failure. Sometimes I feel so angry with my husband I could kill him. I know it's a pride thing. He would feel less of a man if it turned out to be his fault but if he won't co-operate with the doctor, I can't see any way forward. I've threatened everything but he just shuts his ears and then runs round to mummy to get sympathy. I'm seriously wondering if we have a future and we were so happy before all this started.

Dear X,

And you can be happy again but this is quite a serious matter and, yes, your husband isn't being fair to you. The trouble is that he doesn't fully understand the situation. He sees it as a crime not to be able to do what men are supposed to do, father children without any problems. He's indignant that you should think him guilty of that crime and the way forward is to help him understand the true situation. Infertility Network UK, the national infertility support network, can be contacted on 08701 188088 and will provide you with information and support. They will have literature especially aimed at would-be fathers. When he sees that he is not alone and not guilty of anything he should be more amenable.

If not I suggest you contact Relate and get their help in resolving this issue. He runs to mummy because he's hurting like hell and is probably afraid of the future. Arming him with information will make it easier for him to cope and offer you the support and co-operation you deserve.

Dear Denise,
We've had two embryos implanted without
success. They've told me that there was no
reason for them failing but I'm beginning to feel
as though there's something really wrong with
me. Other women seem to find it so easy. I have
a friend who gets pregnant at the drop of a hat.
We laugh about it but actually it's not funny.
I'm beginning to feel really angry and resentful.
Why has this happened to me? Other people have
children they don't value and don't take care of
and I would cherish a child if I ever got one. It's
so unfair. Now I'm wondering if I want to go
through it again when it'll just be a
disappointment. And we can't adopt because my
husband would be classed as too old at 45. I feel
as though the whole family... no, two whole
families... are just watching and waiting for me
to cock it up again. I wish we'd never told them
in the first place and I'd advise any other couple
to keep it all to themselves. Do you think it's
worth another try when that might end in
failure too?

Dear X,

I think giving something important your best shot is always a good idea so I would talk again to your doctors and, unless they tell you differently, think about going ahead. The plain fact is that it is unfair that for some women becoming pregnant is easy and for others it isn't, although you're certainly not alone in that respect. You are entitled to feel angry and I have no words to take away that particular pain. However, if you think about what you are trying to achieve the effort you're having to make should look more worthwhile. Life isn't fair but if you can overcome that unfairness and get the result you want, you will have gone some way to redressing the balance.

As for the families, I understand your annoyance but remember they're watchful because they wish you well. That shouldn't stop you from telling them to back off and give you space but do it gently. I think it would help to talk over your feelings with someone who will understand. Careline in the UK (tel: 0845 122 8622) will lend a sympathetic ear to anyone with a problem. And don't dismiss adoption altogether. It might be possible for you to adopt a slightly older child in the future and that can be an immensely rewarding experience as you restore happiness to a child who has had little enough of it before.

Dear Denise,

I was quite enthusiastic about embarking on fertility treatment but I've changed my mind. My wife has become a fanatic about obeying the rules and increasingly I feel I'm just a tool, a means of her getting what she really wants, a baby. We have friends who've been through it too and they tell me it's two years of hell. I don't honestly think I can take another year of feeling used, even having to come home from work because it's the optimum time and then the eternal wait every month. I'm not with the woman I married, she has become a calculating machine and I feel crushed. Every conversation is about IT, we go to sleep talking about IT and her mother and sister know more about our sex lives than I do. I wish someone had warned me before it began that it takes over and destroys your life.

Dear X,

It's true that the quest for a baby can take over and destroy your life but only if you let it. I sympathize totally with the way you feel and I've heard the story from too many other men to doubt it's true. However, your wife isn't behaving like this on a whim. She is trying to fulfil the agreement you made together and if you can patiently explain that you feel things are getting out of hand, I'm sure she'll try to meet your concerns.

If it's possible, why not take a short break away from routine of all kinds? A few days of remembering you are simply man and woman and not a baby-making machine will do wonders for your morale as long as you both understand beforehand that discussion of the problem is not allowed. Two mad days and nights of enjoyment will bring you back refreshed to take up a routine, which if it's followed, could bring enormous rewards for you both. You've already invested a year of your life, don't let anything spoil things now.

Dear Denise,

I know that time is running out for me as I'm almost 39 but my doctor just tells me to relax and let it happen naturally. Is it possible to talk to a fertility expert without reference from your doctor? I feel he's going to wait until it's too late. We've been trying since I came off the pill a year ago although my husband is away a lot so sex is not always regular. I'm healthy and have never had any gynae problems so it should be alright but it just isn't happening. How long should I wait before I start making a fuss?

Dear X,

I think you're wise to want more information and it might be worth explaining to your doctor that you'd find it easier to relax if you were in possession of more information about future possibilities. He may not have realized how anxious you are and will be more forthcoming about the significance of your age once he understands. Happily there are also organizations that can help. Infertility Network UK, the national infertility support network, can be contacted on 08701 188088 and will provide you with information and support. I wish you well.

10

Your stories

I wasn't prepared for the way getting pregnant would become an obsession.

I always used to think I'd have children one day but if it didn't happen it would be no big deal, I'd have other things in life. Looking back I'm not sure if I really felt like that or if I never properly thought it through.

Anyway, I wasn't prepared for the way getting pregnant would become an obsession the moment I was told it might not be possible. I know that if it never happens we will find other things in life because people just do, don't they? But at times the possibility of failure feels like the end of the world.

Jocelyn

I'm so glad we made the decision to persevere.

We made up our minds to be sensible and see it as the long haul because friends who'd been through it kept saying it might take ages and ages and zillions of tries. In fact, the very first implant took and now I'm like a little whale waddling around. I'm so glad we made the decision to persevere although it was such a shock when it didn't happen once we were trying. It was touch and go whether or not we'd seek help.

Eleanor

I felt like a spare part most of the time.

Now that she's here and I get to feed and change her ... yes, I do change nappies.... I feel ashamed of some of the feelings I had when we were going through it. It was worse for my partner. She was the one that got poked and pulled at. I felt like a spare part most of the time, although, as she reminds me, she couldn't have done it on her own. Anyway, it was worth it.

At the time I used to think it was a bloody waste of time but now I'd go through it again like a shot. Come to think of it we probably will do it again one day.

Robert

I think we'll try for adoption but we're both quite young so there's time to think.

I knew when I looked at him that it wasn't good news. He said we could have another try but it was just as unlikely as the times before. He was lovely all the way through and I really felt he minded as much as we did in the end. We had a bad time for a few months, drowning our sorrows and trying to convince ourselves it didn't matter. And then we got real and started considering options. I think we'll try for adoption but we're both quite young so there's time to think. I don't regret that we tried as hard as we did though. At least we gave it our best shot.

Carolyn

Above all, I couldn't bear the injustice of it.

I've never considered myself a bad person but some of the emotions I felt were frightening. Anger, jealousy ... I resented my sister-in-law because she has babies like shelling peas for Birdseye and she's half my size. Above all, I couldn't bear the injustice of it. We could give a baby everything and other people have them and couldn't care less. Now that we're doing something about it I feel calmer. It's early days but I like the people who are helping us and I'm cautiously optimistic. A woman I work with told me she used to feel the same when she found she was infertile, and showed me a picture of her two kids. It took her a while but it came right in the end. I hope it's the same for us.

Lynda

You always feel it's your decision.

At first the jargon was frightening. We could have done with a medical dictionary, but when we asked them they explained everything in terms we could understand. Now we feel quite calm about it. We're just on the first stage and hoping we won't need to do anything drastic but they don't push you. You always feel it's your decision. I wish our families were the same. Grandmas in search of offspring are scarier than any doctor.

James

Part 5:
More Help
at Hand

11

Keep up the good work

As we enter Part 5 of the book, you are now on the home stretch. We appreciate that there is a great deal of information crammed into these pages and, as we have said throughout, you can revisit relevant chapters as often as it takes to assimilate and digest all the facts we've given you.

Whether you have read the book from cover to cover or you've chosen to cherry-pick the information that is relevant to you at the moment on your fertility journey, this is absolutely fine, as long as you're getting the information and support you need.

In this chapter, we recap on what we know so far and we look at ways for you to continue to help yourselves during what can be a stressful time in your life. In chapter 12, we supply you with contact details for numerous organizations, helplines and websites that you can contact for advice and support. There are also suggestions of other books that you might find useful since we suspect that you will want to read as much information about the subject as possible.

First, let's look at some more ways in which you can get yourself into a positive frame of mind and optimum health for conceiving a baby.

Rejuvenate your mind

We have stressed that a positive approach is highly beneficial when you find yourself facing fertility problems. However, we know it is not easy to simply decide to be positive. So here are a few more strategies that might help you to break out of an old or negative mindset:

Ditch the negativity. Research shows that not only do optimists have better careers and more fun, they are more likely to live to a ripe old age than those who are pessimistic. If your thoughts normally err on the darker side, then challenge yourself! When you catch yourself thinking, 'I'll never have a baby', instead say, 'I'm a healthy fertile woman in optimum condition for conception'. In fact, say it out loud – and defy that negative thinking.

Play to your strengths. When we're doing something we're good at, we feel better about ourselves. Give yourself a chance to shine by building opportunities to do what you're good at into your everyday life.

Surround yourself with inspiring people. Spend time with the people who inspire and excite you rather than those who drag you down

– and keep adding new positive people to your circle – you never know how your world might open up in new and exciting directions.

Try something new. It's good to break your routine and to experience something new and refreshing, from singing to skiing – whatever excites you. Start saying 'yes' when people suggest new things, or make it happen yourself, and this will help to stop your efforts to get pregnant dominating your lives.

Take control. Focus on what you can control and don't worry about what you cannot. For example, you can control what you eat, whether you smoke or drink, your stress levels and how often you have sex, but you can't control whether or not you have blocked tubes, your partner has a low sperm count, or your age. Control what it is within your power to change, and stop worrying about the things that are beyond your control.

Fertility fitness

As you saw in Part 2, Chapter 4, there are certain lifestyle changes that you can make to get yourself into the best possible shape for becoming pregnant. The four cornerstones of this fertility fitness regime are:

- good diet

- plenty of rest

- proper relaxation

- regular exercise.

Here are a few more tips to add to those we've already discussed.

Good diet

The old saying, 'You are what you eat' could not be more appropriate than when you are preparing your body for getting pregnant. So, wherever possible, you want to keep what you put in your body clean, pure and fresh, and this will reap benefits in your general well-being as well as in your reproductive health.

As a general rule, try to choose fresh organic produce and cut down on processed foods with additives and preservatives (cut them out entirely if you're feeling up to it!). Why not stock up on the following, which are known to benefit fertility?

Six of the best

Nuts and seeds provide essential fats and vitamin E, which is sometimes known as the 'fertility vitamin' because it carries oxygen to the sex organs. Brazil nuts, in particular, are also a good source of selenium, which is important for protecting sperm and egg health.

Kiwi fruits and oranges are a great source of vitamin C, which helps to maintain the quality of sperm and eggs.

Green leafy vegetables, such as broccoli, spinach and kale, are a great natural source of folic acid, which is essential to a developing embryo.

Whole grains including brown rice are rich in B vitamins, zinc, manganese and selenium as well as fibre.

Water – try to drink bottled or filtered water because tap water can contain lead, pesticides, oestrogens, chlorine and other toxins that impair fertility.

Shellfish are an important source of zinc, which is essential for healthy sperm production as well as cell renewal and repair.

Foods to avoid or cut down on

Liquorice – studies have shown that liquorice can decrease testosterone levels in men, contributing to impotence or sexual dysfunction.

Coffee and tea cause further anxiety or stressful symptoms in the body.

Artificial sweeteners, particularly aspartame, have been linked to infertility and miscarriage. These are usually found in 'diet' or 'sugar-free' foods and drinks, so it pays to read labels.

Alcohol – the effects of alcohol on fertility have been discussed in Chapter 4 and it should be avoided as much as possible while trying to conceive and throughout pregnancy.

Hydrogenated fats – recent studies indicate that hydrogenated fats (also known as trans fats) reduce fertility in both men and women. Again, try to get into the habit of reading food labels – or better still, avoid processed foods altogether wherever possible.

A good night's rest

If you are stressed or anxious about becoming pregnant, it's a good bet that you're not sleeping well. Unfortunately, this can become a vicious circle because lack of sleep makes you more tired and anxious, and also depresses your sex drive – none of which helps when trying to conceive. Here are a few tips for a good night's sleep:

Six of the best

1 Have a muscle-relaxing warm bath at bedtime, and why not add a couple of drops of lavender or rose oil which are known to be soothing?

2 Sip herbal tea such as valerian (great for calming an over-active mind) or chamomile (a natural sedative) before going to bed.

3 Have a bowl of porridge. Sounds odd, but oats are an excellent nerve tonic and the milk contains tryptophan, an amino acid produced by the brain, which helps regulate sleep (hence the reason why people also like to have a milky bedtime drink).

4 Listen to calming music and make the bedroom a tranquil haven rather than a cluttered mess.

5 Avoid stimulants such as coffee, tea, alcohol and chilli during late evening.

6 If you can't get to sleep, try not to panic. Instead, use the relaxation technique we describe below to relax your muscles and mind.

Proper relaxation

In Chapter 4, we looked at various ways of dealing with stress, which is the enemy of fertility, from breathing techniques to visualization. Don't forget to keep practising these skills, and here is another great exercise that you might like to try for relaxing the body and calming the mind.

1 Either sit comfortably or lie down.

2 Close your eyes and take one or two calming breaths.

3 Starting with the feet, you are going to work your way through the body, clenching and

then relaxing the muscles. So, tightly clench your toes and then gently uncurl them.

4 Then, in slow progression, clench and release:
   – calves
   – thighs
   – buttocks
   – stomach

5 Now, screw your hands into a tight fist and then relax the hands and let them drop.

6 Hunch your shoulders up tightly, hold for two to three seconds, and then let them drop.

7 Pull your face into a tight scowl, hold for two to three seconds and then release and let your face relax.

8 Take a couple of deep breaths and then slowly open your eyes. The tension should have slipped away from your body and you should feel calmer and more relaxed.

Gentle exercise

In the Western world, most are guilty of leading sedentary lives, but as you saw in Chapter 4, exercise can help to maintain a good weight which is important when trying to get pregnant, and it can generally improve health and vitality.

Although it is important that you make time for exercise, this doesn't mean you have to go to the gym. There are other ways of building more exercise into your lives, such as using stairs rather than lifts and walking short distances rather than taking the car, all of which can help.

However, taking up an activity, such as swimming, cycling or running, is great if you can fit it into your busy schedule. Or why not kill two birds with one stone by considering one of the Eastern arts such as yoga or Tai chi? These condition the body but are also great for relaxing the mind.

To give you a taste of what you might expect, here is a basic yoga pose (āsana) that is great for flexibility but also strengthens the back and pelvic area and revitalizes the whole body. If you suffer from back, neck, wrist or knee pain, consult your doctor before trying the exercise.

The cat (Bilikāsana)

- Kneel on all fours with your hands shoulder width apart and your knees the same distance apart as your hands.

- Your arms should remain straight throughout the entire exercise.

- Breathe out while arching your back up high. Keep your head between your arms, looking towards your abdomen.

- Hold this pose for a few seconds.

- Breathe in as you slowly hollow your back to a concave position.

- Raise your head and look up. Hold again.

- Repeat the sequence five times, creating a slow, flowing movement between the two postures. Take your time

- Relax.

Moving on

You've just about reached the end of the book but, of course, this is not the end of the road. For many of you, it's just the beginning. We hope that all the information we've given helps you to navigate a way through what may have appeared like a minefield at the outset. Hopefully, you are now feeling more confident about the options that are available and about what choices might be right for you. We also trust that, as you've moved through the book, we have been able to answer your questions and settle many of your concerns. However, if you have any questions left unanswered, then we provide a whole host of different sources and organizations in Chapter 12 that will undoubtedly have experts on hand to help you with your specific query. Please don't be afraid to approach these organizations; they are very accessible, keen to help and sympathetic to all those who are seeking more information and assistance on fertility issues.

You know now that you are not alone. There are many other couples all over the UK who are also experiencing difficulties in conceiving. They understand what you are going through and they are available in support groups and in online chat-rooms and forums to share their experiences and to support and empathize with you.

What now?

Some of you may have already embarked on fertility investigations and even treatment, in which case, we hope things are going well for you and that our book is of some help or comfort. For those who are still at the stage of assessing your options, evaluating your goals and raising questions, the information and suggestions in the book are designed to help you to put together a plan that seems best suited to you and your partner.

Whatever you decide, whether you wish to change your lifestyle and carry on trying on your own, or you opt for tests and assisted conception techniques, there is no right or wrong decision. We are confident that you will make the best choice for your unique situation in the light of how you are both feeling at this moment in time. This is a journey – plan as much as you can but, remember, **you can always revise what you want** as new information comes to light.

Wherever you find yourselves on your fertility journey – whether deliberating your choices, waiting for test results or preparing for treatment – we urge you to keep eating healthily and to take time to relax and chill out. Try to be kind to yourself and to each other. You have already been through a lot and you may have more challenges to face. Wherever possible, make an effort to offer and accept love and support from your partner, friends and family through the months to come.

We understand that dealing with fertility problems can be a difficult and demanding experience. Whatever the outcome, whether you reach your goal of having a baby or whether you embrace a childfree future, the experience can make you stronger, more independent and more self-aware. It can also strengthen your relationship and bring greater understanding, love and respect to your partnership.

If you can manage to stay positive and hopeful throughout your fertility journey, and see beyond your difficulties at each step along the way, then you will have done remarkably well and you should be justifiably proud of yourselves. Perhaps most importantly, don't forget to keep talking to one another – you and your partner are in this together and, as a team, you will overcome your fertility issues.

Finally, we hope more than anything else that your dreams are fulfilled. Good luck.

12

Helpful organizations and further information

General

Careline
Helpline: 0845 122 8622 (Monday to Friday 10 a.m. to 1 p.m., 7 p.m.–10 p.m.)
UK national confidential telephone counselling service.

National Institute for Clinical Excellence (NICE)
Tel: 020 7067 5800
www.nice.org.uk
Independent organization responsible for helping patients to make decisions about treatment and health care.

NHS Direct
Tel: 0845 4647
General advice on health matters from the UK's National Health Service.

Samaritans
Tel: 08457 90 90 90 (24 hours).

Infertility

Ashermans Syndrome
www.ashermans.org

Assisted Conception Babies (AceBabes)
Tel: 0845 8381593
www.acebabes.co.uk
Support for families following successful fertility
treatment.

British Fertility Social Secretariat
22 Apex Court
Bradley Stoke
BS32 4JT
Tel: 01454 642277
www.britishfertilitysociety.org.uk
Representing those who work in reproductive
medicine.

**British Infertility Counselling Association
(BICA)**
69 Division Street
Sheffield S1 4GE
Tel: 01744 750660
www.bica.net

Childlessness Overcome Through Surrogacy (COTS)

Tel: 0844 414 0181

www.surrogacy.org.uk

Information on implications of surrogacy through experiences of others.

Daisy Network Premature Menopause Support Group

www.daisynetwork.org.uk

Members can speak to others who have been through egg donation cycles.

Donor Conception Network

PO Box 7471

Nottingham NG3 6ZE

Tel: 020 8245 4369

www.dcnetwork.org

Ectopic Pregnancy Trust

Tel: 01895 238025

www.ectopic.org

Endometriosis SHE Trust (UK)

14 Moorland Way

Lincoln LN6 7JW

Tel: 08707 743665/4; **www.shetrust.org.uk**

Endometriosis UK
50 Westminster Palace Gardens
1–7 Artillery Row
London SW1P 1RR
Helpline: 0808 808 2227
www.endo.org.uk

**Human Fertilisation and Embryology
Authority (HFEA)**
21 Bloomsbury Street
London WC1B 3HF
Tel: 0207 291 8200
www.hfea.gov.uk

Infertility Network UK (INUK) (formerly
CHILD and ISSUE which merged)
Charter House
43 St Leonards Road
Bexhill-on-Sea TN40 1JA
Tel: 08701 188088
www.infertilitynetworkuk.com

The Miscarriage Association
c/o Clayton Hospital
Northgate, Wakefield WF1 3JS
Helpline: 01924 200799
www.miscarriageassociation.org.uk

More to Life
Infertility Network UK
Charter House
43 St Leonards Road
Bexhill-on-Sea TN40 1JA
Daytime advice line: 08701 188088 Mondays,
Wednesdays and Fridays (10 a.m.–4 p.m.)
www.infertilitynetwork.uk.com
Support for the involuntarily childless.

National Gamete Donation Trust (NGDT)
PO Box 2121
Gloucester GL19 4WT
Tel: 0845 226 9193
www.ngdt.co.uk

Polycystic Ovary Syndrome Support Group (VERITY)
22–24 Highbury Grove
London N5 2EA
www.verity-pcos.org.uk

Progress Educational Trust (PET)
140 Gray's Inn Road
London WC1X 8AX
Tel: 020 7278 7870
www.progress.org.uk

Provides information on assisted reproduction and human genetics.

Stillbirth and Neonatal Death Society
28 Portland Place
London W1B 1LY
Helpline: 020 7436 5881
www.uk-sands.org

Surrogacy UK
PO Box 24
Newent GL18 1YS
Tel: 01531 821889
www.surrogacyuk.org

UK Donorlink
31 Moor Road
Headingley
Leeds LS6 4BG
Tel: 0113 278 3217
www.ukdonorlink.org.uk
Voluntary register following donor conception pre-1991.

Women's Health Concern
PO Box 2126
Marlow SL7 2RY
Tel: 01628 488065
www.womens-health-concern.org

Useful websites

These sites give you an opportunity to ask questions and exchange personal experiences with others:

www.fertilityfriends.co.uk
www.may-b-baby.co.uk
www.gettingpregnant.co.uk
www.ivf-infertility.com
www.mindbodyfertility.co.uk

Adoption and fostering

Adoption Matters
14 Liverpool Road
Chester CH2 1AE
Tel: 01244 390938
www.adoptionmatters.org

Adoption UK (previously PPIAS)
46 The Green
South Bar Street
Banbury OX16 9AB
Tel: 01295 752240
Helpline: 0844 848 7900
www.adoptionuk.org

Adults Affected by Adoption – NORCAP
112 Church Road
Wheatley
Oxfordshire 0X33 1LU
Tel: 01865 875000
www.norcap.org.uk

Barnardo's Children's Charity
Jigsaw Project
12 Church Hill
Walthamstow E17 3AG
Tel: 020 8521 0033
www.barnardos.org.uk/jigsaw

**British Association for Adoptions
and Fostering (BAAF)**
Saffron House
6–10 Kirby Street
London EC1N 8TS
Tel: 020 7421 2600
www.baaf.org.uk

Independent Adoption Service (IAS)
121–123 Camberwell Road
London SE5 0HB
Tel: 020 7703 1088
www.i-a-s.org.uk

Intercountry Adoption Centre (also Overseas
Adoption Helpline)
64–66 High Street
Barnet EN5 5SJ
Tel: 0870 516 8742
www.icacentre.org.uk or www.oah.org.uk

Jewish Association for Fostering, Adoption and Infertility (JAFA)

PO Box 20, Prestwich
Manchester M25 5BY
Tel: 0161 773 3148

National Fostering Network

87 Blackfriars Road
London SE1 8HA
Tel: 0207 620 6400
www.fostering.net

Overseas Adoption Support & Information Services (OASIS)

20 Woodland Terrace
Greenbank
Plymouth PL4 8NL
Tel: 0870 241 7069
www.adoptionoverseas.org

Post-Adoption Centre (PAC)

5 Torriano Mews
Torriano Avenue
London NW5 2RZ
Tel: 020 7284 0555
Adviceline: 0870 777 2197
www.postadoptioncentre.org.uk

Useful website

www.adoption-net.co.uk

Complementary therapies

Association of Reflexologists
27 Old Gloucester Street
London WC1N 3XX
Tel: 0870 5673320

British Acupuncture Council
63 Jeddo Road
London W12 9HQ
Tel: 020 8735 0400
www.acupuncture.org.uk

British Association for Nutritional Therapy (BANT)
27 Old Gloucester Street
London WC1 3XX
Tel: 08706 061284
www.bant.org.uk

The British Homeopathic Association
Hahnemann House
29 Park Street West
Luton LU1 3BE
Tel: 0870 444 3950
www.trusthomeopathy.org

British Hypnotherapy Association UK (BHA)
Tel: 020 7723 4443
www.british-hypnotherapy-association.org

The Institute for Complementary Medicine
Tavern Quay
Plough Way
London SE16 7QZ
Tel: 020 7237 5165
www.i-c-m.org.uk
Provides information on complementary
medicine and administers the British Register of
Complementary Practitioners.

The Society of Homeopaths
11 Brookfield
Moulton Park
Northampton NN3 5WL
Tel: 0845 450 6611
www.homeopathy-soh.org

Counselling

British Association for Counselling and Psychotherapy (BACP)
BACP House,
35–37 Albert Street,
Rugby CV21 2SG
Tel: 0870 443 5252
Email: bacp@bacp.co.uk
www.bacp.co.uk
Contact this organization for details of local counsellors and therapists (fee paying).

British Confederation of Psychotherapists (BCP)
(a.k.a. British Psychoanalytic Council)
West Hill House
Swains Lane
London N6 6QS
Tel: 020 7267 3626
www.bcp.org.uk

Careline
Helpline: 0845 122 8622 (Monday to Friday
10 a.m.–1 p.m., 7–10 p.m.)
UK National confidential telephone counselling service.

Relate
Herbert Gray College
Little Church Street
Rugby CV21 3AP
Tel: 0845 456 1310 or 01788 573241
www.relate.org.uk
Relationship counselling.

Depression

Aware
72 Lower Leeson Street
Dublin 2
Tel: 01 661 721
Helpline (loCall): 1890 303 302
www.aware.ie
Organization to assist those whose lives are directly affected by depression.

Depression Alliance
Helpline: 0845 120 3746 (weekdays 7 p.m.–10 p.m.)
www.depressionalliance.org

Depression Alliance Cymru (Wales)
Tel: 029 2069 2891

Depression Alliance Scotland

Tel: 0845 123 23 20

www.dascot.org

Fellowship of Depressives Anonymous

Box FDAI

c/o Self-Help Nottingham

Ormiston House

32–36 Pelham Street

Nottingham NG1 2EG

Offers information, support, and local groups.

Mind

15–19 Broadway

London E15 4BQ

Tel: 020 8519 2122

Information line: 0845 766 0163

www.mind.org.uk

The English national association for mental health, which has many local branches.

No Panic

93 Brands Farm Way

Randley

Telford TF3 2JQ

Free helpline: 0808 808 0545 (every day, 10 a.m.–10 p.m).

www.nopanic.org.uk
Information and support for panic attacks,
phobias, obsessions.

Samaritans
Tel: 08457 90 90 90 (24 hours)

SANE
1st Floor Cityside House
40 Adler Street
London E1 1EE
Tel: 0845 767 8000
www.sane.org.uk

**United Kingdom Council for Psychotherapy
(UKCP)**
2nd Floor
Edward House
2 Wakley Street
London EC1V 7LT
Tel: 020 7014 9955
www.psychotherapy.org.uk

Preconception

Foresight (Association for the Promotion of
Preconceptual Care)
178 Hawthorn Road
West Bognor PO21 2UY
Tel: 01243 868001
www.foresight-preconception.org.uk

Pregnancy

National Childbirth Trust (NCT)
Tel: 0870 770 3235
www.nctpregnancyandbabycare.com

Useful books

The Baby Void, My Quest for Motherhood, Judith
    Uyterlinde (Summersdale)
*Fertility and Conception – The Complete Guide to
    Getting Pregnant* – Zita West (Dorling
    Kindersley)
*Fit for Fertility – Overcoming Infertility and
    Preparing for Pregnancy*, Michael Dooley
    (Hodder & Stoughton)

In Pursuit of Parenthood: Real-life Experiences of IVF, Kate Brian (Bloomsbury)

PCOS and Your Fertility: Your Essential Questions Answered, Colette Harris with Theresa Cheung (Hay House)

The Subfertility Handbook, Virginia Ironside and Sarah Biggs (Sheldon Press)

Swimming Upstream, David Rawlings and Karen Looi (Landmark Media)

Understanding Infertility, Peter Wardle and David Cahill (The British Medical Association)

Dealing with emotions

Banish Anxiety, Dr Kenneth Hambly (Thorsons)

Depression: The Way out of your Prison, Dorothy Rowe (Routledge)

Fatherhood: The Truth, Markus Berkmann (Vermilion)

How to Improve your Confidence, Dr Kenneth Hambly (Sheldon)

Living with Stress, Cary Cooper (Penguin)

Managing Anger, Gael Lindenfield (Thorsons)

Overcoming Stress, Dr Vernon Coleman (Sheldon)

GLOSSARY

Abortion Termination of a pregnancy, either spontaneously by the body or induced through medical intervention prior to the twentieth week.

Aesthenospermia *See 'Low motility'*

AI *See 'Artificial Insemination'*

Assisted reproductive technology (ART) The collective name for all artificial techniques used to assist conception.

Adhesions Scar tissue formed by the body following surgery, infection or disease.

Amenorrhea Absence of periods.

Amniocentesis A diagnostic procedure performed by inserting a hollow needle through the abdominal wall into the uterus and withdrawing a small amount of fluid from the sac surrounding the foetus. It's used to detect chromosomal disorders such as Down's syndrome, structural defects such as spina bifida, and other rare, inherited disorders.

Anovulation Absence of ovulation.

Antenatal Prior to birth. Also called 'prenatal'.

Areola The area surrounding the nipple.

Artificial insemination (AI) A process where the sperm of a donor male (husband or unknown) is inseminated into a woman's vagina, cervix or uterus.

ART *See 'Assisted reproductive technology'*

Aspermia There is no ejaculation.

Azoospermia The absence of sperm in male ejaculation.

Cervix The narrow neck at the lower end of the uterus or womb that joins the vagina.

Chlamydia A bacterial sexually transmitted disease that can damage the male and female reproductive systems.

Chorionic Villus Sampling (CVS) A prenatal test (during pregnancy) that is used to detect chromosomal defects.

Clomid (clomiphene citate) A drug used to induce ovulation.

Conception The fertilization of an egg by a single sperm to create an embryo.

Cryopreservation The freezing of gametes or embryos.

CVS *See 'Chorionic Villus Sampling'*

Cyst A fluid-filled sac. Often found in the ovary where it does not contain an egg.

Dilation and curettage (D&C) A procedure where the interior of the uterus (womb) is scraped to diagnose a disease or to clear out uterine contents. Often used after a miscarriage.

Donor insemination (DI) The introduction of donor sperm into the cervix or womb.

Dysmenorrhea Painful periods.

Ectopic pregnancy A pregnancy that implants outside the uterus, for example, in the fallopian tubes, abdomen, cervix or ovaries.

Egg The female gamete released during each monthly menstrual cycle (period).

Egg collection The removal of eggs from a woman's ovary after stimulation during in vitro fertilization (IVF) using either a laparoscope or an ultrasound-guided needle.

Egg donation The donation of eggs by a fertile woman for use in fertility treatment.

Egg sharing During the course of in vitro fertilization (IVF) treatment, a woman uses some of her eggs but also donates some for others to use.

Embryo A fertilized egg that has the potential to develop into a foetus.

Embryo freezing A process in which 'spare' embryos are frozen and stored for future use.

Embryo transfer The transfer of embryos into the female patient.

Endometrium The lining of the womb (uterus) which sheds during menstruation and which supports a foetus when pregnancy occurs.

Endometriosis The abnormal growth of endometrial tissue outside the uterus.

Epididymus A coiled tube that connects the testes to the vas deferens, through which sperm travels.

Fallopian tube(s) The tube where the egg and sperm meet that links the ovaries and the womb.

Fertile You are fully capable of conceiving and sustaining a pregnancy.

Fertility Ability to produce children.

Fertility drugs Hormones used in fertility treatment.

Fertilization When a sperm successfully penetrates into an egg, forming an embryo.

Fibroid A non-cancerous (benign) grown that is found in the uterus.

Fimbrioplasty Surgical procedure to peel back the blocked end of fallopian tubes.

Foetus A developing embryo after eight weeks of development until birth.

Follicle A small sac in the ovary in which the egg develops.

Follicle-stimulating hormone (FSH) A hormone released from the pituitary gland that stimulates follicle production. It is also used in assisted conception to stimulate the production of several follicles.

Gamete A sperm or egg.

Gamete Intra-Fallopian Transfer (GIFT) An assisted-conception procedure in which eggs are retrieved, mixed with sperm and replaced back into the fallopian tube for fertilization to take place naturally.

Gonadotrophins Reproductive hormones (follicle stimulating hormone and luteinizing hormone) from the pituitary gland.

hGC *See 'Human chorionic gonadotropin'*

HFEA Human Fertilisation and Embryology Authority.

Hormones Chemical messengers produced by various glands. Also made synthetically to mimic actions of natural hormones.

HSG *See 'Hysterosalpingogram'*

Human chorionic gonadotropin (hGC) The presence of this hormone in female blood or urine indicates a pregnancy.

HyCoSy (hysterocontrastsalpingograpy) An assessment of the fallopian tubes using ultrasound to look for blockages

Hyperstimulation Over-stimulation of the ovaries following super-ovulation drug treatment.

Hysterosalpingogram (HSG) An X-ray of the fallopian tubes to detect any obstructions.

ICSI *See 'Intra-cytoplasmic sperm injection'*

Immotile Used to refer to sperm that don't swim or move.

Implantation Where an embryo embeds itself in the lining of the uterus.

Impotence A man's inability to produce or sustain an erection.

In vitro fertilization (IVF) Fertilization of the egg by the sperm outside the body in laboratory conditions (prior to being replaced in the womb or frozen).

Infertile If you have been having unprotected sex for over 12 months (six months if you are a woman over 35 years old) without conceiving naturally, then you are considered infertile by the medical profession.

Infertility counselling Specialist counselling on the medical, ethical and emotional implications of infertility treatment.

Intra-cytoplasmic sperm injection (ICSI) A procedure in which a single sperm is injected into an egg.

Intrauterine insemination (IUI) Insemination of sperm into the woman's uterus.

IUI *See 'Intrauterine insemination'*

IVF *See 'In vitro fertilization'*

Laparoscopy An internal examination of the abdomen and pelvic area using a telescope inserted surgically through the abdomen (usually under general anaesthetic).

Low motility (aesthenospermia) The sperm are unable to wriggle and move as they should, even if the sperm count is normal.

Low sperm count (oligospermia) There are some sperm present but not as many as normal.

Luteinizing hormone (LH) Hormone secreted in the pituitary gland. It is essential for the development of eggs and sperm.

Menstrual cycle A woman's monthly cycle occurring over approximately 28 days, where an egg is released from the ovary and the womb lining prepares to receive the egg (if fertilized) or to shed it via the vagina (if not fertilized).

Mucus hostility Condition where a woman's cervical mucus kills off her partner's sperm before it gets a chance to swim up the cervical canal to reach the egg.

Multiple pregnancy A pregnancy of two or more foetuses.

Myomectomy Surgery to remove fibroids.

Normospermia Normal semen analysis.

Oestrogen Female hormone produced by the ovaries. The levels of the hormone change during the menstrual cycle.

OHSS *See 'Ovarian Hyperstimulation Syndrome'*

Oligozoospermia (oligospermia) Low sperm count.

Oocyte Female egg (gamete)

Ovarian Hyperstimulation Syndrome (OHSS) A serious complication following the stimulation of the ovaries using ovulation-induction drugs.

Ovarian stimulation Stimulation of the ovaries to produce eggs, either when the ovaries are underactive or, in assisted reproductive technology (ART), to cause super-ovulation (extra egg production) artificially.

Ovary The female reproductive organ that contains and releases eggs.

Ovulation The monthly release of the egg from the ovary triggered by a surge of luteinizing hormone.

Ovum Mature egg (plural: **ova**)

Parabens A group of preservatives widely used in cosmetics that mimics the hormone oestrogen.

PCO *See 'Polycystic ovaries'*

PCOS *See 'Polycystic ovarian syndrome'*

Pelvic inflammatory disease (PID) Infection of the female organs within the pelvis. This can lead to scarring and adhesions in tubes, contributing to sub-fertility. This is the most common cause of female infertility.

Percutaneous epdidymal sperm aspiration (PESA) Retrieving sperm directly from the epididymis using a needle.

Peritoneum The thin lining that covers all the organs of the abdomen.

Phytoestrogens Naturally occurring compounds that mimic oestrogen and are hormone-balancing.

PID *See 'Pelvic inflammatory disease'*

Polycystic ovarian syndrome (PCOS) A condition that can lead to irregular periods, excessive hair, acne and infertility, among other symptoms.

Polycystic ovaries (PCO) A common condition where ovaries increase in size with small cysts. PCOs may lead to polycystic ovarian syndrome (PCOS).

Post-coital test A test performed on the sperm and cervical mucus after intercourse to check for mucus hostility and sperm survival.

Premature menopause A condition where a woman ceases to ovulate and has her menopause before the age of 40.

Progesterone Female reproductive hormone secreted by the ovary and corpus luteum to mature the lining of the uterus for conception, and during pregnancy.

Prostate gland Male gland that contributes a major portion of the fluid that makes up semen.

Salpingitis Inflammation of the fallopian tubes following infection.

Salpingogram X-ray of the fallopian tubes.

Salpingostomy Surgical operation to open the fallopian tubes near the ovary end.

Secondary infertility Cases of infertility where a pregnancy has previously occurred and a child or children have been born.

Semen Fluid of the male ejaculate including sperm and other secretions.

Semen analysis Test for sperm motility, morphology (appearance) and density.

Sperm Male gametes. A single sperm is called a 'spermatozoon'.

Sperm bank Clinic where donors give sperm and where it is stored.

Sperm count *See 'Semen analysis'*

Spermatid An immature sperm cell.

Spontaneous pregnancy A pregnancy achieved without artificial reproductive technology (ART).

Sterile Permanently infertile.

Sub-fertility A problem, not necessarily untreatable, which inhibits conception.

Surrogacy The use of another woman to carry a baby and give birth to it for a woman who cannot sustain a pregnancy. This can involve embryo implantation or it may involve the use of surrogate's eggs inseminated by the male partner of the couple.

Teratospermia The semen contains a high number of abnormal sperm (sperm with split heads, no tails and other abnormalities).

Testes Testicles or male gonads.

Test-tube baby Popular term for a baby fertilized in vitro, literally meaning 'in glass'.

Testosterone The male hormone (women have a small amount of this hormone too).

Transvaginal aspiration Method of egg recovery in which a needle is inserted into the ovary.

Transvaginal oocyte recovery Method used to retrieve eggs using a needle that is passed through the vagina under ultrasound guidance.

Treatment cycle One complete treatment.

Trimester Pregnancy is divided into three phases, known as trimesters. The first lasts from conception to week 12, the second ends at 28 weeks, and the third encompasses the rest of your pregnancy until birth.

Tuboplasty A surgical procedure to open blocked fallopian tubes.

Ultrasound (ultrasound scan) A diagnostic device that uses sound waves rather than X-rays to examine the body. This can be done on the abdomen or vaginally.

Unexplained infertility Cases where no pathological reason can be found in either partner yet pregnancy isn't occurring.

Uterus The womb, where the embryo develops.

Vaginismus A condition where the muscles around the vaginal opening contract in spasms making intercourse painful or impossible.

Varicocele A varicose vein on the scrotum/testes.

Vas deferens The tubes that link the epididymis to the urethra and transport the sperm.

Vasectomy Surgical tying of the vas deferens to produce voluntary sterilization.

Xenoestrogens Artificial chemicals that, due to their chemical structure, act like oestrogen in the human body.

Zygote A fertilized egg.

Zygote Intra-Fallopian Transfer (ZIFT) Similar to GIFT (Gamete Intra-Fallopian Transfer), except fertilized embryos are transferred to the fallopian tubes while the woman is under general anaesthetic.